GESUNDHEIT!

GESUNDHEIT!

**Bringing Good Health to You,
the Medical System, and Society
through Physician Service,
Complementary Therapies,
Humor, and Joy**

PATCH ADAMS, M.D.
with Maureen Mylander

Healing Arts Press
Rochester, Vermont

Healing Arts Press
One Park Street
Rochester, Vermont 05767
www.InnerTraditions.com

*Note to the reader: This book is intended as an informational guide. The remedies, ap-
proaches, and techniques described herein are meant to supplement, and not to be a substitute
for, professional medical care or treatment. They should not be used to treat a serious ailment
without prior consultation with a qualified healthcare professional.*

LIBRARY OF CONGRESS CATALOGING-IN-PUBLICATION DATA

Adams, Patch, 1945–
  Gesundheit! : bringing good health to you, the medical system, and
  society through physician service, complementary therapies, humor,
  and joy / Patch Adams ; with Maureen Mylander.
      p. cm.
  Includes bibliographical references and index.
  ISBN 0-89281-781-X
  1. Physician and patient. 2. Gesundheit Institute. 3. Community
  health services—West Virginia. 4. Medical care, Cost of—United States.
  5. Health reformers. I. Mylander, Maureen. II. Title.
  R727.A32 1992
  362.1'01—dc20   92-7008
                                                                    CIP

Printed and bound in Canada

10 9 8 7 6 5 4

This book was typeset in Palatino with Kabel and Goudy as the display typefaces

Page 27: Patch with watering can. Photo by Ben Stechschulte.
Page 117: Patch with children. Photo by Ben Stechschulte.
Pages 164, 165,166: Exterior, entrance, and ground plan of Gesundhei Hospital.
Illustrations by Dave Sellers
Pages 168, 169,170: Eye clinic, ear clinic, and hospital equipment. Illustrations by
    John Connell. E-mail: connell@madriver.com

Healing Arts Press is a division of Inner Traditions International

Dedication

To Anna Hunter, my mom, who gave me the foundation for everything I like in myself.

To Linda, who was there from the beginning, working hard for the dream and who had the tenacity to cope with me for twenty-six years, and to J.J., Gareth, Kathy, Blair, and Heidi, without whose devotion and help this dream would never have happened.

Contents

Publisher's Preface

When Universal Studios expressed interest in making a movie about Patch Adams and *Gesundheit!* we at Healing Arts Press couldn't have been more delighted. From the time the *Gesundheit!* manuscript first arrived in our office we have been avid fans of Patch and his band of healer-clowns, and of the true spirit of life and love they bring to their work. Their inspiring vision of a different sort of medicine and their unflagging belief in a dream that too many shortsightedly called "impossible" has won respect and admiration, not only from us but from people the world over. It is a testament to Patch's conviction and tenacious determination that he has never abandoned his quest, and that he continues to help and to heal people, as well as to believe that his dream for a new paradigm of medical treatment—a free hospital—will soon become a reality.

In December of 1998 Universal Studios is releasing a film version of Patch's life, starring Robin Williams, bringing this important story to an international audience. It seems only fitting that an actor of such unique comic and dramatic talents as Williams should be chosen to play Patch. It is easy to see these two men as kindred spirits, two individuals who are blessed with the ability to make us laugh and who enrich the world around them through the generous expression of their gifts.

Thousands of readers have been moved by the story of Patch's life and work and his dream to build a hospital that uses laughter as a form of medicine, love as its currency, and trust and acceptance as the very bricks of its foundation. We at Healing Arts Press hope that this film and the new exposure it gives to the story of *Gesundheit!* will prove the catalyst that finally brings to Patch and his friends the support, recognition, and success they deserve.

Foreword

I nauthenticity is our modern form of plague: it kills life.

The human essence of fundamental relationships is obscured by procedures, technology, and regulations. Eight-second sound bites drive political processes; our families become the focus of justice as the right of children to divorce their parents is affirmed; a Norwegian M.I.T. student is "punched out" to death by a trio of high school students seeking excitement. We are out of touch with the historic roots that give our lives meaning.

So, too, in health care we are out of touch with what gives us meaning. At a time when the power of our technology makes possible undreamed-of interventions in the diseases of mankind, the very relationship between doctor and patient has become a battleground. Distrust and disrespect prevail where alliance and intimacy are most needed. What we as physicians have lost in this process is almost too much to acknowledge: the dreams that guided us into a profession combining Hippocratic diligence with Samaritan obligation.

Patch Adams is an unlikely wake-up call for us. Soon after meeting him, I realized that this Clown was deadly serious. His Clowning has the power of all good humor: to reveal to us what we have become and to do so in a mood of good humor that allows us to see.

In this book, Patch returns us to what we have forgotten:
• That all of us are humans and as such inhabit our own stories—the historic traditions that make each of us unique, not just a "case." In fact, each patient's traditions not only are contained in

the uniqueness of this moment, to be listened to and savored, but are integral to the generation of the suffering and healing of this particular human. Listening, not just hearing, is central. The Clown says, "when we gave up house calls, we gave up the gold."

• That we, the doctor and patient, stand a better chance of making it through life's darkest moments as intimate and respecting partners, not in hierarchical roles. Enough of the white coats, and the teams of house staff swooping to the bedside to talk of the "gall bladder" that was admitted last night. The Clown introduces himself to his patient while riding a unicycle.

• That life itself is bigger than illness, diagnosis, treatment, or disease mechanism. A moment of laughter, a walk in the country, simple touching, or tears can reorganize biology in a way that drugs cannot. The Clown builds a hospital with a farm and a drama theater.

• That humility is essential. He reminds us that we are mortal, that death is always in the background, and that if we take ourselves in passionate—but not ponderous—significance, we can have more fun than we have now and be at least as effective. For the Clown, humor, celebration, gratitude, and invention are all crucial elements.

So, readers, both professionals and patients (in the end, we are all patients), ready yourself for a joyful shock as you read these pages. Let yourself dream about how life could be, and be inspired into action by someone who has the courage to live his dreams.

Matthew A. Budd, M.D.
Assistant Professor of Medicine
Harvard Medical School
Director of Behavioral Medicine Programs
Harvard Community Health Plan
Cambridge, Massachusetts

Author's
Acknowledgments

I had wanted to defer writing this book until after our new hospital in Pocahontas County, West Virginia, had been open for two years. I envisioned a do-it-yourself book on how to take a huge dream from its initial spark to its final reality: a dream-weaver's manual. The high demand for our ideas and plans, sparked by my lectures and correspondence, has brought this book out early. We are also hoping that the book will help trigger the financial thrust necessary to complete our dream hospital.

Let me pour out precious thanks to:

My coauthor, Maureen Mylander, without whom this book would not have happened. She took the raw material from interviews and many essays and has created a cohesive book. Her solid belief in its value has sustained me.

Ehud Sperling of Inner Traditions for believing in our work and for being persistent.

My mom and my brother, Wildman, who were my major sidekicks in life well into my medical career.

Mary Ann Kernecklian, who, for several years before I wrote the initial paper about Gesundheit in March 1971, spent many evenings with me helping me find myself and define my values, encouraging my idealism, and believing in my abilities.

Clare Shumway, who now looms as the doctor at Medical College of Virginia and who, by his example, most strongly influenced my becoming the kind of doctor I wanted to be.

Gareth Branwyn, who for ten years has been my right hand in

creating the ultimate dream hospital. Living with you, in thousands of sizzling hours of dialogue, has been ecstatic. So much of our direction has come from your intelligent, creative suggestions.

J. J., probably the single strongest influence on my sustained commitment to Gesundheit. Your friendship and devotion to our crazy dream is intoxicating. I am so glad you and Eva Bear came together. Her devotion to the dream and willingness to be the assistant director have taken a tremendous administrative burden off me.

And the "zanies," that amorphous mass of silly humanity that became the pilot experiment where we tested our ideas and ideals for Gesundheit. You are my inspiration to continue. I salute you, especially those of you who lived with me and gave up your privacy to be in so many people's lives. We had a glorious adventure together. This new hospital will thrive because of what you taught me.

And finally, Linda, Zag, and Lars, my family, my anchors: wherever I have gone these twenty-plus years, you have been there. Thank you for your love and fun, for you are the most intense and amazing experiment of all!

Patch Adams, M.D.

Coauthor's Preface

The first time I saw him, he was wearing a rubber nose, a multi-colored print shirt, and a polka-dot tie over yellow balloon pants held up by suspenders. Beneath the rubber nose was an elaborate handlebar mustache; on the back of his head, a ponytail that reached to his waist. He stood before an audience of Maryland hospital administrators who snickered at first, then smiled, then fell silent, and ended up thunderously applauding and inviting him to their regional conference.

Meet Hunter D. "Patch" Adams, M.D., a social revolutionary and one-man show, who believes in "horse and buggy" medicine and never charges his patients a cent! Patch has become a celebrity in medical circles because his ideals—and his plans for transforming them into reality—kindle the hope of rediscovering the joy in practicing medicine, for health care professionals and patients alike.

We decided to collaborate on a book about a unique and positive approach to health and healing. It tells, in Patch's voice, how he and a few colleagues came to found the Gesundheit Institute in Northern Virginia in 1971. During the next twelve years, they operated a fun-filled, home-based family medical practice and managed to see more than 15,000 people without bills or other compensation, malpractice insurance, formal facilities, and other "necessities" of modern medicine.

Patch believes that healing should be a loving, creative, humorous human interchange, not a business transaction. Today's high-tech medicine has become too costly (thus he doesn't charge or use third-party insurance), dehumanized (he spends up to four hours taking

each patient's initial history), mistrustful (he refuses to carry malpractice insurance), and grim ("Good health," he says, "is a laughing
matter.").

Our book, *Gesundheit!*, is about hope and humanism in medicine. The
introduction describes the practicalities of how Patch and his colleagues
came to create an alternative health care facility—the Gesundheit
Institute—and how Patch's ideals led to this stunning result.

Part I presents Patch's philosophy of how to make people feel better
and draws on dozens of his most popular essays. Patch writes about
burnout, third-party insurance, malpractice, alternative therapies,
house calls, and cure rates. He explores humor as an antidote to all ills.
His writings on friendship and community explore the effects of
boredom, loneliness, and fear on health and happiness. From "How to
Be a Nutty Doctor," to "Nasal Diplomacy" and "Fun Death," these
writings present the core values of the Gesundheit Institute and its
unique approach to health and healing. They are also a prescription for
personal and professional happiness. What if they caught on?

Part II presents the blueprint for Patch's dream of a forty-bed free
hospital on 310 acres in a medically underserved area of West Virginia. The Gesundheit Institute, in its new home, will be open to
"anyone from anywhere."

Patch has told his story in hundreds of speeches, on radio, and in
TV appearances over the past decade at colleges, churches, corporations, community groups, and medical schools and conferences. He
has intrigued audiences who have wanted to know *more*. And in the
process, he has become something of a media event as he uses humor
and showmanship (clowning, walking a slack rope, riding a unicycle)
to get his points across. A Patch presentation in 1985 touched off a
clowning crusade on the Harvard Medical School quad that brought
smiles to the faces of passersby and brought patrons of the Windsor
Bar out on the street. One of them said, "You guys are gonna be
doctors?! That's great!!"

This positive vision of the future addresses the concerns of millions of Americans who, public opinion polls consistently show, are
unhappy with—and increasingly hurt by—deficiencies in our health
care system. Exposure to this sane but wacky voice will inspire the
medical community and people who are searching for hope and
optimism about their health and that of future generations.

Maureen Mylander

Introduction

Health is based on happiness—from hugging and clowning around to finding joy in family and friends, satisfaction in work, and ecstasy in nature and the arts.

When a dream takes hold of you, what can you do? You can run with it, let it run your life, or let it go and think for the rest of your life about what might have been.

Gesundheit Institute is the dream of a growing number of people, an experiment in holistic medical care based on the belief that one cannot separate the health of the individual from the health of the family, the community, and the world. We have taken the most expensive service in America, medical care, and given it away for free. We are now building a facility in West Virginia that embodies this philosophy: a free, home-style hospital and health center, open to anyone from anywhere. We want this center to be a health care model, not necessarily to be copied by others but to stimulate caregivers and hospitals to develop an ideal medical approach for their communities.

One of the most important tenets of our philosophy is that health is based on happiness—from hugging and clowning around to finding joy in family and

1

friends, satisfaction in work, and ecstasy in nature and the arts. For us, healing is not only prescribing medicine and therapies but working together and sharing in a spirit of joy and cooperation. Much more than simply a medical center, the Gesundheit facility will be a microcosm of life, integrating medical care with farming, arts and crafts, performing arts, education, nature, recreation, friendship, and fun.

Yes, we want the world to change. Gesundheit Institute is a sociopolitical act that has grown out of a deep concern for the quality of people's lives in a world dominated by the values inherent in greed and power. Health care is at a crisis, just as family life and community are in crisis. We don't want to be a Band-Aid for ailing health care; we want to change the system, to bring about a peaceful revolution. We hope this book will be seen not as the definitive answer but rather as a stimulant to big dreams and big actions. The more we spread the word about our work, the more we help others rethink the system, the more powerful that revolution will be.

Growing Up Gesundheit

A man needs a little madness, or else he never dares cut the rope and be free.

Nikos Kazantzakis, *Zorba the Greek,* the film

In view of the direction my life has taken, it may seem an improbable beginning: I was born an Army brat, into an institution that both cares for and controls people as they practice to conduct warfare. The Army also gave me a sense of what the rest of the world is like, and it allowed me to develop social skills as I moved from place to place: Germany for seven years, Japan for three, and Texas, Oklahoma, and many other places for briefer periods. I learned to make new friends quickly because weeks or months later they—or I—would have to move whenever our fathers were ordered to assume another duty.

I always did well in school, especially in math and science. Smart kids often aren't stimulated enough in school, and their response is to act out. I made trouble not by being violent or breaking things but by being a verbal troublemaker: questioning the rules, acting like the class clown.

After school, my friends and I shot a lot of pool. This was a very important part of my life until I went to college. I was a good pool player because I am mathematically inclined, and I enjoyed figuring the angles of incidence and refraction. I even made some money at it. I also challenged myself by playing difficult solitaire games until I mastered them.

Being an A student in math and science made life seem easy and gave me another solitary pursuit. I remember getting a microscope for Christmas when I was about twelve and spending months gazing at a new universe of life forms, each intoxicatingly unique. Next I rushed to explore chemistry. I was living in Germany at the time and could go to local apothecaries to buy any chemicals and laboratory equipment I wanted. In my upstairs laboratory, I dissected animals and conducted all kinds of experiments. I remember keeping stale fish blood—I can smell it still—in a test tube. I would open it and "odorize" the room whenever I wanted to explore science undisturbed. Mathematics, the mother of all the sciences, enchanted me. It was so perfect and so gloriously orderly that I spent day after day delving into the smallest details.

I don't remember when or why science and math began to dominate my interest. I loved exact, rational problems that, however complex, had distinct answers. Word puzzles and mechanical puzzles occupied me for hours, even days. This love of order trickled into my personal life as a penchant for cleanliness and organization.

In the seventh grade, when we were living in Kaiserslautern, I started entering science fairs. One entry involved dissecting a frog for the judges (it won first place at the All-Europe science fair); another involved keeping a guinea pig's heart alive in Ringer's solution, a substance that was physiologically close enough to blood to sustain "life" in the form of a beating heart.

In the third year, determined to make it to the All-Europe competition again, I created a project that I was sure would win. I decided to study gibberellin, a plant hormone that could make cabbages grow twelve feet tall and make flowering plants mature remarkably quickly. I had read about the project in a science magazine and knew that very little work was being done with this hormone in Germany. So I chose this subject not so much because of my interest in gibberellin as to impress the judges. The strategy succeeded. I won first place in biological science for a project called "The Effect of Gibberellin on Economic Crops." I don't remember my father's reaction, but my mother was thrilled.

My mom was the rock of my childhood. My father, an Army officer in the infantry and artillery, wasn't at home much, but my mother lavished love and attention on us. She had a great sense of humor and was always interested in learning new things. Most of the good in me came from my mother. My older brother, Robert Loughridge Adams, known as Wildman, was my sidekick during much of my youth. We decided to be close so that whatever else changed, we would always have each other.

Soon after that last science fair, my father died suddenly. I was sixteen; it happened right after I had spent a week alone with him. My mother and brother had been away, I had just started my first job, and he suddenly asked me to take several days off work. I'm sure that psychics would say that he had some premonition he was going to die and that this awareness made him bare his soul to me in a way he never had before. While I was growing up, he was away most of the time and generally just sat in a chair and drank when he was home. Whenever we asked him about the wars he'd fought in, he would start to cry.

But during that week we spent together, he told me how World War II and the Korean War had destroyed his spirit. Today it's called post-traumatic stress syndrome, a condition that went totally unrecognized and uncared for in those and previous wars. The Korean War was far more devastating to him than World War II because issues of right and wrong were not as clear in Korea. Even worse, his best friend had buried a grenade in his own stomach to save my father's life. My dad felt guilty about that and about never having been wounded. But the greatest guilt of all involved his family: he apologized to me for not having been a good father.

Just as I finally became friends with my dad, I lost him. He had come home from World War II with undetected heart disease and high blood pressure. At the end of that week in 1961 when we finally connected as father and son, he suffered a heart attack. Soon after the ambulance took him away, we called the hospital for news of him. He died within half an hour, with no family around him and no chance to say good-bye. To this day, I feel angry and cheated that I was not with him.

The three years that followed were the most tumultuous of my life. My mother, my brother, and I were uprooted from Germany, our home of seven years, and catapulted into the civilian life of suburban northern Virginia, my mother's home. We lived with my aunt and uncle for several months before settling into a place of our own. My uncle was a wonderful man, a lawyer and an independent thinker in a society of conformists. He was generous and fun, and he cared for me. We played chess together. He loved gadgets and showed me how they worked. He quickly became my surrogate father. Even after we moved to our own house, I spent many hours talking to my uncle. He was a good listener and a superb storyteller.

A few months after my father's death I was still suffering but couldn't express my feelings, either to my mother or to myself. She had been brought up with the attitude "If it's unpleasant, don't talk about it." Rather than mourn, I fought the system. At the high school I attended in Arlington, Virginia, I stood up against segregation and prejudice and developed a reputation as a "nigger lover." I went to sit-ins and marches. Religion offered no solace and felt hypocritical to me, and I turned against it; I would seek out people who believed in Christianity and try to crush their beliefs because they had no proof. In school I became increasingly rebellious; although I was in the math honor society, my teachers wouldn't recommend me for the National Honor Society because of my defiant attitude. I didn't care.

My mother had gotten a job as a teacher and gave us all of her love and support, just as she always had. But even with her great love, I was no longer a happy person. Science and reason had been my solace in the past, but I could no longer find enjoyment in the inexhaustible mysteries of nature.

I turned to writing articles against segregation, religious hypocrisy, and war. (The antiwar articles came in handy later in establishing my conscientious objector status with the military.) I also wrote poems about the pain I was feeling. One began, "Weary am I and full of despair that moves me through this iced chill. . . ."

When I wasn't fighting the system, I was trying to escape it. I wanted to go out with girls but they weren't interested in me. When they turned me down for dates, I would think how shallow and stupid most high school girls were for going out with what seemed like dumb athletes. Since I couldn't get dates, I joined the jazz club, which consisted of three other guys—all nerds. Sipping beers in Washington clubs, we heard some of the hottest jazz musicians of the 1950s and 1960s. I went to coffeehouses and listened to "beat" poetry. And I shot a lot of pool.

By the end of November of my senior year, I started having pains in my stomach. The X-rays revealed ulcers, and my doctor prescribed the traditional remedies: bland diet, medication, and milk. My book bag was stuffed with Gelusil and half-and-half, and my pockets with Librium and Rubinol, which made me sleepy all the time. The ulcers recurred the following spring, and I was hospitalized a second time. I was literally eating my guts out. My mother wouldn't talk to me about anything unpleasant, and I had nobody else to notice that I was deeply troubled: no confidant, no mentor of great wisdom, no father. I didn't know what to do with my life—whether I was going to the freedom marches or to college, or whether I would even live.

At the beginning of my freshman year in college, Donna, my girlfriend from senior year of high school, broke up with me. The uncle I had adopted as a surrogate father committed suicide. I flew home to his funeral and a few weeks later dropped out of school. A pulsing inner chant told me to die without hope. Once I took twenty aspirins, thinking that would kill me. I obsessed about suicide every day but needed to work up to it, so I went to a cliff near the college called Lover's Leap and sat at the edge, writing epic poetry to Donna. I composed sonnets, searching for the right words that would really get to her. If I had ever finished my outpourings I would have jumped; fortunately, I was too long-winded.

After a disastrous visit to Donna, during which I tried to lay a guilt trip on her, I took a Greyhound bus home and trudged six miles through the snow to my mother's doorstep. When my mother opened the door I told her, "I've been trying to kill myself. You'd better check me into a mental hospital." She called the family doctor, who called a psychiatrist, who admitted me to a locked ward at Fairfax Hospital. I spent Halloween there. My two-week stay was the turning point in my life. The people who had the greatest impact on my recovery were not doctors but my family and friends, especially my roommate, Rudy.

Rudy had had three wives and fifteen jobs and lived in an unfathomable abyss of failure and despair. When my friends came to visit me, I realized how good it felt. But nobody ever came to visit Rudy. He told me about a loneliness I had never dreamed existed, and that made my pain seem trivial by comparison. For the first time in my adult life, I empathized with another person.

Talking to Rudy, I realized the importance of love and the people who loved me. I had been surrounded by love but hadn't let it affect me. I perceived a deep personal truth: I needed to be open to receive love. Without it I was not a strong person. And I realized that if I continued living as I had been—without tender, human love—I would end up like Rudy. He represented the Ghost of Christmas Future that I would become if I refused to surrender to my needs.

That moment was a spiritual awakening to the power of love. My destructive use of science, math, and reason to disprove whatever was not factual had, in fact, left me very lonely. I talked to the other patients on the ward and found similar threads of loneliness and lost dreams. It became obvious, through the tears, that these people weren't crazy or insane. There was no switch in our heads for "normal" or "abnormal." I was the same person I had always been; so were they. Maybe that's what was so painful. These supposedly "crazy" people had merely responded to life's complexities with fear, anger, sadness, and despair to such an extent that they—we—needed protection from ourselves.

I saw a very significant movie about that time: *Zorba the Greek*. My dilemma was the same as that of the English bookworm in the story. "You think too much, that is your trouble," Zorba told him. "Clever people and grocers, they weigh everything." I stopped thinking that *thinking* mattered more than anything else and started putting feelings first. After ten or twelve days in the hospital, I told my mom, "I'm all right now," and she believed me. She had never acknowledged that I needed to be in a mental hospital in the first place. "You're not crazy," she said. And she was right in the sense that I was a soul in pain, not insane. The psychiatrist thought I should stay longer, but I wanted to leave and signed out against medical advice.

The most important influences on my life so far had been my dad's death, having a great mom, and going through an illness at an early age. Hospitalization had forced me to formulate a philosophy about happiness. A new experience began that affects the way I am today: I became—for want of a better word—a student of life, of happy life. My initial forays into the human condition during hospitalization expanded. I wanted to know everything possible about people and happiness and friendship, so I turned to the centuries of wisdom as captured between the covers of great books. I read all the works of Nikos Kazantzakis, the author of *Zorba*. I read books written by Nobel laureates in literature, including Jean-Paul Sartre, Thomas Mann,

William Faulkner, and Bertrand Russell. I also read Plato, Nietzsche, Dostoyevsky, Balzac, Franz Kafka, Charles Dickens, Walt Whitman, Virginia Woolf, Ayn Rand, Emily Dickinson, and many more classics of nineteenth- and twentieth-century fiction. Whenever I heard a book mentioned three times, I'd buy and read it. Like many others who have suffered, I became tremendously interested in what I had gone through. The world of the arts helped me understand my new fascination with living humankind.

My best "bibliography" grew out of my personal interactions with people. I wanted to know what made them feel good and sought out happy families so that I could understand what glued them together. I experimented with friendliness by calling hundreds of wrong numbers just to practice talking to people; I wanted to see how long I could keep them on the line and how close we could get. I'd pretend to be a sociology student, or an artist, or anything that would help me draw people out and get them to talk to me. I went out in public and engaged strangers in conversation. I rode elevators to see how many floors it would take to get the occupants introduced to one another, and even singing songs. During the summer between my second and third years of college, I went to local neighborhood bars several nights a week and didn't allow myself to leave until I knew—or had tried to learn—everybody's story. I could scarcely believe how great and unique people were, yet how common the threads of their stories. Like a modern Ancient Mariner, I felt compelled to talk to everyone possible about life and its joys and woes. I became an explorer of continents of experience and fun, a journalist who didn't keep notes.

I was becoming an intentional person, experimenting with new behaviors in a methodical way. At last science had come back into my life, this time fortified by faith in friendship, with human beings as the experimental subjects. I'm still that kind of scientist, always doing research in the laboratory of humanity.

After leaving the hospital, I knew I wanted to perform some service and decided to go into medicine. I applied for the premedical curriculum at the George Washington University in Washington, D. C. My acceptance was delayed because the admissions people wanted me to take eight or nine months to see psychiatrists and get myself together. While waiting to be admitted, I worked in Anacostia, a neighborhood of Washington, as a file clerk.

The file room of the Navy Federal Credit Union in Anacostia might seem like an unlikely place to thrive. The people who worked there spent half their waking hours doing something they hated. Filing was considered particularly horrible work: joyless, boring, and dull. I decided to change all that. My fellow file clerk was Louis Fulwiler, who remains my oldest friend. Louis, like me, had dropped out of college temporarily. From the very first day we decided to make the files a "happening"—it was, remember, the mid-1960s—and egged each other on. We drove to and from work wearing kids' aviator helmets with little noisemakers that went "vah-roooooorrrr." We interacted with other people in the office by singing file information. One day, when anybody asked us for a file, we replied in a high-mass Gregorian chant, "Which file do you wa-ant?" Another day we arrived for work attired in gorilla suits. Louis was my partner in fun, and we gave each other the courage to be goofy in public. When we went back to visit ten or fifteen years later, everybody still remembered us. We had opened whole new vistas in the filing shtick.

This early foray into the world of humor and fun encouraged me to expand and get better at it. I always could find an audience, even at the 7-Eleven. I discovered that fun is as important as love and life. The bottom line, as I had noticed during my phone conversations with strangers, was that when I asked people what they liked about life, they described the fun they had, whether it was racing cars, playing golf, or reading books.

Nurtured by levity and love, I blossomed. I defeated all my demons and became the person I am today. My self-confidence, love of wisdom, and desire to change the world were rooted in that brief period, from late 1963 to fall 1964, when I climbed out of despair to rebirth.

I entered pre-med school in the fall. As an undergraduate I lived with my mom and attended classes at George Washington University, coming home every day to study. I did a huge amount of reading beyond my college assignments, particularly of the great works of literature that would help me understand more about the human condition. For fun, I continued learning to be a silly person. This was the period when I called most of the wrong numbers to practice getting to know people. My scientific side said, "How are you going to learn about people unless you talk to a lot of them?" To better understand different facets of society, I went to Ku Klux Klan and Black Muslim meetings. I became more involved in civil rights and started thinking about bigger and bigger social issues. Our involvement in Vietnam, well established by then, hung like a dark cloud over socially conscious students like me.

When I entered medical school in 1967, I didn't know much about medicine; I just expected to become a doctor without realizing what that meant. I soon found out. The Medical College of Virginia in Richmond is a very conservative state school. No blacks were admitted in my class, and the school establishment favored the Vietnam War. Both policies were totally repugnant to me. Fortunately, I had developed a strong sense of myself and knew that I wanted to get my medical degree and serve society. My role models of devoted and caring service were Albert Schweitzer and Tom Dooley.

Almost from the outset, I found that many of my professors were aloof, arrogant, and devoid of any vision of a humane health care system. The emphasis was on the patient as a passive recipient of wisdom, which demigods handed down from a temple of technology. Patient advocacy and consumerism were unheard of.

The tragedy was that we students were subtly squeezed into a mold that to me seemed inhumane. Hospital staffs were not designed to work together as teams to relieve suffering. Doctors supposedly knew all the answers and ordered others around, often rudely. This kind of thinking—the doctor as a hero who saves the patient—is destructive because it instills the belief, in students and everybody else, that the doctor has all the answers. There was no room for humility or mistakes. What pressure this put on students of medicine! We quickly learned that malpractice lawsuits were a likely reward for trying to help others. We learned the politics of buck-passing and the gymnastics of cover-up when the inevitable mistakes were made. We learned of doctors who invested heavily in the companies that served their patients. We stood in the shadows that greed—perhaps society's greatest ill—casts over the field of medicine.

Reductionism dominated in classes and on the wards. People were called by the names of their diseases, as if the disease were more important than the human who suffered from it. We were taught to ask the patient quick, penetrating questions in order to ascertain which tests to order and which medications to prescribe. We learned to gather this vital information in five or ten minutes at the most. All other facets of the patient's life—family, friends, faith, fun, work, integrity, nutrition, exercise, and much more—were considered virtually irrelevant to medical practice. Most discouraging of all, patients seemed endlessly willing to submit to this approach. In fact, whenever one dared to question a physician's action or decision, he or she invariably was labeled a "problem patient."

During my freshman year the school offered an optional three-hour course called "Man and His Environment." The professor made a great effort to introduce us to the many complexities of life and health care situations outside of the hospital. Only 20 to 40 percent of my classmates signed up, and the next year the class was dropped. The whole idea of a person's life—its quality, diversity, and complexity—was relegated to psychiatry. But the psychiatry texts did not discuss any aspects of a healthy, happy life, much less suggest how to attain it. Instead, they were filled with descriptions of pathology and case histories of bizarre mental disorders. On the psychiatric rotation, conversations between doctors-in-training and patients—when they occurred at all—conveyed all the uptight tension of the Victorian era. There was no friendliness or laughter, and God forbid we should have ever talked in an enlightened way about sex. To this day, whenever I tell people I'm interested in a person's life, joys, woes, and family, they say, "Oh, you're a psychiatrist!"

Joylessness prevailed not only on the hospital wards but in the classrooms as well. Many of my professors conveyed a total lack of excitement about the field of medicine. By and large, they didn't seem to like lecturing and were not very good at it. They had to lecture in order to keep their university positions, but their true interest was research.

In reaction to the prevailing atmosphere, I wrote a manifesto and hung it on a wall at the medical school. This is an edited version:

I came to medical school on two legs, but left on four wrapped in wool. . . . The school emphasized how we looked, not how we act. . . . They gave us an image. We ironed it right in, stay-press. We carry it around with us to impress our friends, better still, our patients. Patients, patients, my God, we'd forgotten about them. A few paid, but we had to turn most of them away. A guy's got to live, you know: yachts, golf, sustenance. So we finished, yes, and joined the AMA and parted ways. You know something funny, someone said that no one commits suicide like doctors. How could that be? Now we're professionals with prestige, money, title, nothing.
(Signed) X Person

After two years of academics, we moved on to learn medicine in the hospital wards. This was even more disturbing than the classroom phase. By that time, I realized that most people—including many health care professionals—suffered from the same emptiness, loneliness, and boredom described in the works of great literature I had been reading. They were leading lives of quiet or noisy desperation.

Already I had decided that I didn't want to live this way. I was learning about medicine but avoided making my medical school experience a misery as many of my colleagues were doing. Since the academic aspects of medical school weren't especially difficult for me, I experimented with sports for the first time and joined the Richmond Rugby Club. To keep myself from burning out, I took off at least one day a week and most of the weekends and probably dated more than at any other time of my life. For the first time, women found me attractive. Perhaps it was partly because I didn't care which residency I would get. My goal wasn't Harvard or Yale, so I wasn't playing that game. I asked the school administration not to notify me of my grades unless I was failing.

The best fun of all was interacting with patients. I rebelled against grand rounds and the impersonality of ten strangers in white coats trooping into a sick person's room. The air of solemnity was so thick that I preferred to visit patients when the heavies weren't around. I discovered that if I entered a hospital room and was vibrant and smiley, the patient would immediately perk up. At 6'4" tall, with long hair, a mustache, and a black patch safety-pinned to the lapel of my white jacket to call attention to the Vietnam War, I looked different from most of my colleagues. I discovered that the patients were thrilled to have me there. I was free to talk to the patients, cry with them, massage them, comfort them, joke with them, and inject some exuberance and fun into their lives. My initial appearance sometimes gave them pause, but a friendly personality won them over.

The patients loved it. The nurses loved it. My fellow students were another story: some loved it and some hated it. Many were threatened by me. A hospital was supposed to be very serious: people were suffering and dying, and doctors should be solemn. But I didn't want that. Sometimes, of course, solemnity was entirely appropriate, but most of the time it was not.

My professors responded, predictably, in the idiom of the haircut. The powers-that-were emphasized how we looked, not how we behaved, and they wanted us to look alike: short hair, three-piece suits, and no facial foliage. They didn't care whether or not we were humanists. I also clashed with my professors about keeping a professional distance. Getting close to the patients was forbidden because it might lead to transference—emotional involvement—or a lawsuit. Yet I had felt the magic each time patients freely offered their vulnerability and trust. It felt natural to sit beside them, open myself to the same vulnerability, and share my life with them. My professors objected to this closeness, to my sitting on the bed with patients or massaging their feet. "You get too involved," they said.

One of the best programs at the Medical College of Virginia offered the opportunity to spend the entire senior year pursuing individual interests through elective courses. My interest was pediatrics, so I chose to spend from September 1970 to March 1971 at a children's clinic in a ghetto in Washington, D. C. The clinic was affiliated with Children's Hospital and headed by Dr. Peg Gutelius. Her compassion and sense of humor created a relaxed, friendly atmosphere: my kind of setting. I was given full responsibility and freedom to spend time with the children. I was allowed to bring friends in and paint cartoons all over the walls. In short, I was encouraged to be myself.

I had played the role of Santa Claus in the past for retarded children and those in Head Start programs, so I appeared at the clinic in my Santa suit. The kids immediately called me "Dr. Ho Ho." Every day was a thrilling new experience, but the greatest thrill was provided by the healing environment and the team effort to help children and their families. Most of the patients had no funds to pay for our services and no other way to get help, so the clinic had the flavor of free medical care with a smile. I loved it.

During the same period, I spent fifteen hours a week at the Free Clinic in the Georgetown area. This hippie-style clinic was open at night and was run by volunteers. Here medicine was practiced with the sole intent of relieving suffering—shoestring medicine with yard-sale décor. What an emergency room! People came from all over the Washington area and beyond: some dressed to the nines and some in fraternity garb, street people, hippies playing guitars and singing, others passing out leaflets for a cause, suburban teenagers seeking birth control pills, drug users, "soldiers" of the antiwar underground, people worried that they would catch something just by being there, curiosity seekers, and many more. They sat or stood together in one room, with piles of clothing in one corner, blankets for whoever needed them in another, salads and a pot of fortifying beans in a third. People brought useful items to share with others. The walls were covered with posters, placards, and 3" x 5" cards describing lost relatives. A lot of medicine—the most gratifying kind—was happening there, allowing each practitioner to be his or her best self.

The Free Clinic offered an ideal environment in which to experiment with humor and see whether it could help others. One day I wore a fire hat and a red rubber nose to work and discovered that my nuttiness did not diminish the respect or trust of the patients. In fact, it seemed to enhance these feelings. Humor helped me become closer to many of the patients. I spent lots of time with them and was invited on occasion to their homes. The closeness that resulted from spending time together was indistinguishable from friendship. This was the context in which I wanted to work: friendship enhanced by a sense of no indebtedness. I found myself loving to be at work and went there on my nights off. This facility and the children's clinic provided the models for what I wanted to do with my medical career.

My training had brought me face to face with the American medical system. I knew I would have difficulty finding room for myself in it. Where does a happy-go-lucky person go? Where does service-oriented medicine go? To an Indian reservation with huge rolls of red tape? To pediatrics? Are these the only choices? Some of my colleagues quit medicine because of such incompatibilities. One was so burned out that he became a ski instructor. Most of them just stayed in medicine and gave up their original ideals. I kept on doing what I thought was right. By my last year I had become quite vocal, not realizing that my actions would be seen by my school as a threat.

The last weeks of medical school were soured by a clash with an assistant dean, who threatened that I wouldn't graduate. He criticized me in a memo as being "excessively happy." The dean's office even frightened my mother with fabricated stories about irresponsible behavior on my part. I had planned to wear my Santa suit to graduation, but this experience so embittered me that I refrained.

To counterbalance this low point of my medical school experience, two good things happened. One was that I met Linda Edquist, a tall, beautiful "child of the sixties," who has been my friend, companion, and wife since that time. She was a volunteer in the adolescent clinic where I spent my last two months in training. For our first date, I took her to a balloon party, something I'd dreamed about doing for many years. I filled my apartment with balloons from floor to ceiling. With twenty or so people in the room, no one could see anybody else, but whenever one person moved, everybody could feel it. It was a circus of sensations and a very interesting date for her—and for me. Attracted by her independence, generosity, and playfulness, I said to myself, "My God, what a delicious woman." She went back to the dorm and told her friends, "I just had the strangest date of my life. I think I'm going to marry this guy."

The other positive thing was that when I returned to the Medical College of Virginia for the last three months of my final year, I began working on a line of thought that would shape the rest of my life. I still planned to go into pediatrics and spent many hours reading about education, believing that a pediatrician should be familiar with the subject. I thought that if I could be a children's doctor in a school and become involved with the students and their families, maybe the general health of the students would improve. I wrote letters to schools proposing this idea but got no response. Finally, I realized that if I had dreams about improving health care, I would have to carry them out myself.

My mind was ablaze with alternatives. A group-communal situation seemed the most promising approach; I had read extensively on utopian philosophy and had visited the Twin Oaks commune in Virginia in 1969. But I knew of no models in America for a therapeutic medical community that put humanism first. I was concerned that the legal constraints on conventional medical practice would never permit such an experiment.

I still intended to complete a pediatric residency and work with children and teenagers, but I decided to design another model. For six weeks I toyed with many ideas. Finally I drew up a grandiose plan—having no idea how grandiose at the time—that I felt ready to commit myself to. I wrote it up in one night, not really knowing how serious I was or how my ideas about an ideal medical facility foretold the rest of my life's work.

Titled "Positive Thinking," the plan was about providing health care in the best interests of patients and staff alike. I envisioned a community where people with poor self-images could go, actively participate in rebuilding their lives, and reestablish love of self and of others—the most potent therapy of all. I envisioned a farm of about 75 to 100 acres with a primary school, a library, dormitories for as many as 300 patients, and facilities for artists, craftspeople, and other skilled individuals drawn from America's alcoholics. We would have gardens to make the community self-sufficient and a range of projects—such as building tree houses—to make work a joyous game. The community would have a permanent staff of doctors and health care professionals and a temporary staff of teachers and other helpers. Most people would stay only a few hours or days, but those needing the community for longer periods would stay longer. "Communication, both verbal and nonverbal, will be our way of life," I wrote.

> *Much of this dream is sketchy, but rigidity will be frowned upon and spontaneity rewarded. Love of self, others, the environment, and life will be our by-products, not through proselytizing, but through experiencing life as a joy. When a child is born, he is placed in a world of war, apathy, and competition, where self-assertion and individuality are discouraged, and love of others and of life is felt to be fantasy. We will have a community where joy is a way of life, where learning is regarded as our greatest aim, and love as the ultimate goal. . . . We will not call it a dream, but will live it as a reality.*

This statement meant that I had decided partly to work with the system and partly to change it, rather than show how stupid the system was. The dream started with the abstraction of wanting to give service and evolved through different forms into a bold new proposal for health care delivery. The model had no name at first; not until 1979 did we name it the Gesundheit Institute. We chose the name because it makes people laugh, and thus become open to healing, and because literally translated, Gesundheit means "good health."

Preparing for Gesundheit

My residency at Georgetown University Hospital was like returning to the Dark Ages: to the burnout of medical school and to the huge numbers of "physically healthy people" whose lives were miserable. I was looking for an environment like the children's clinic, where levity and love prevailed. What I found in the pediatric department at Georgetown University Hospital approached the other extreme.

Medical procedures, often painful and traumatic, were overused at the expense of spending time observing and talking to patients. For example, at the time it was customary to perform a spinal tap on all children with convulsions, even though the convulsions often were no more than reactions to a high fever. In my view, intuition and time spent observing young patients could have prevented most of those painful, traumatic procedures. As another example, private physicians often admitted children with diarrhea or vomiting to the hospital when called by first-time, inexperienced, frightened mothers, and then administered intravenous fluids, when empathy and support, not hospitalization, more often were needed.

I decided to quit the residency (the staff at Georgetown acknowledged my incompatibility quite graciously) and become a family doctor. I set up my practice at home, a three-bedroom house I shared with some friends in Arlington, Virginia, where I could express freely my ideals of loving patients and using humor and fun as therapy.

The Pilot Project

That first communal experiment grew into twelve years of practicing medicine from our home, a caring environment where play and shared experiences were as important as the medical treatments. In various locations, from Arlington, Virginia, to farms in West Virginia, we lived what was in effect a pilot program for our dream of a free, full-scale hospital and health care community. We never charged our patients or accepted payments through health insurance. We refused to carry malpractice insurance. We practiced as we saw fit, emphasizing preventive medicine and welcoming alternative therapies. An acupuncturist set up practice in our basement, and we began to allow other practitioners—homeopaths, chiropractors, naturopaths—to see patients at our house. It was a stunning hive of activity and a most exciting time in my life.

In September 1973, two years after I finished medical school, Linda and I, with thirteen others who had been working together, toured Europe for eleven months in a royal blue, 1952-vintage bus. We spent this time exploring human closeness and all the ways we could make our relationships tight and solid.

The intimacy and openness we developed on this trip were important for the next stage of our work. First in Fairfax County, Virginia, and next in Jefferson County, West Virginia, twenty of us lived and worked together. We farmed, kept goats, and explored play in many forms. In any given month, hundreds of people would visit us, drawn by word of mouth. They would come either for medical care or to participate in the activities with which we explored the enriching potential of play. Some who came for social activities—craft fairs, plays, dances—came back later for medical help. Treatment of patients took place in the course of daily life as we took walks, did the dishes, or played together.

We served patients who traveled great distances for medical treatment as well as healthy people who wished to formulate a prevention program. Their "office visits" lasted from a few minutes to five months. Patients with chronic medical problems that had not been solved by traditional healing methods, as well as those who were overwhelmed by the side effects of their treatments, came to us hoping to find alternatives. They inspired us to search for solutions that had been condemned in our medical training. We studied medical history and alternative medical literature. In the hope of finding respite for those who continued to suffer, whether from "real" or "imagined" illnesses, we sought out people who had solved their problems outside allopathic methods. Time after time, we found testimonials of cures or alleviated symptoms. We asked specialized health care professionals to treat selected patients under our supervision. To our great surprise and delight, many patients were helped by alternative therapies. These new approaches became a wonderful addition to our allopathic treatments.

During those twelve years, we discovered that most patients needed much more in their lives than medication. Health seemed interwoven with an individual's perception of quality of life. Often, dissatisfaction with work, family, and self prevented a "cure" or improvement in health from ever happening. It seemed imperative that we understand how to prevent or alter these tragedies if we were to address each person's health problems effectively. These issues traditionally have been the province of philosophy, psychology, the arts, and religion, so we studied each of these areas extensively.

When I saw a patient, I would spend hours learning about his or her parents, lovers, friendships, jobs, and hobbies: the entire person. This vastly expanded version of the traditional—and often truncated—"patient history" was the only way we could learn what affected a person's health and build a relationship between us. Most patients didn't want the level of intensity that I was willing to give, but any degree was better than nothing. I believe that my patients got what they came for and that their eyes were at least partially opened to the healing power of intimacy.

I have never defined people by their diseases. Most individuals in our society are unhappy about their lives and need a huge amount of psychological and spiritual nourishment. Suppose a person with cancer came to me and we spent 100 hours together. How many of those hours would we spend talking about the physical aspects of the cancer? Two hours, or maybe ten. The rest of the time, we'd talk about the human being and why it would matter whether that person lived or died. How long could I talk about the pain in someone's joints? The patient could describe it. I could do a physical exam. I could prescribe acupuncture, or homeopathy, or pills. And that's it. But that person might still have the pain.

People sometimes ask, "What were your cure rates?" This question is predicated on "cases" in the classical medical sense of "six cases of diabetes," "five cases of heart disease," and so on. We didn't have *cases* of disease. We saw individuals with medical problems or needs. I kept minimal records but estimated that the flow of people through our facility was 500 to 1,000 a month. There were no waiting rooms. Never did we say, "This person's here for X-ray," or "That one's here for lab work." *Being* there was the therapy. To us, medicine was—and is—the relationship between healer and patient. So whether someone visited to work in the garden, drop by for dinner, or just see what was happening, our goal was to build a solid relation-ship. It was a slow process. Many of our patients had seen other doctors, often quite a few doctors. They had described signs and symptoms. The doctors had run tests and prescribed a treatment or two, and that was their relationship. It often required a long, long romance to impart an alternative vision of what the doctor–patient relationship could be.

Since all this occurred in our home, we considered it paramount to our own health to have an environment that was loving, humorous, creative, cooperative, and open to change. We operated an organic farm, a wide variety of arts and crafts projects, and a recreation program. An important part of our health message was that people need people. We felt that many people could lessen their anxieties and loneliness if they were supported by strong friendships, families, and community systems.

We tried in our personal lives to be examples of how this could happen. Usually we were a staff of fifteen to twenty people, including at least two physicians and often more, in a suburban farm setting. We lived together under one roof, virtually forgoing our private lives. Each staff person played many roles: farmer, cook, mechanic, clerk, nurse, doctor, artist. Our learning to live cooperatively and happily inspired many of our patients to seek closer community ties after returning home.

Moving On: Publicity and Fun(d)-raising

In 1979, I stepped back from our work in order to reflect on our ultimate goal: building a hospital where we could carry out our commitment to free health care. This step was prompted by the frustration of several people in the project who, after eight years, had had enough of sacrificing their private lives and struggling for a dream that never seemed to come closer. We were then living at The Rocks, a farm in West Virginia. Linda and I moved closer to Washington to concentrate on fund-raising and a limited medical practice; the people who remained at The Rocks ultimately stopped providing medical care but have remained together as a community.

Fund-raising was slow until 1983, when we decided to abandon twelve years of media silence and actively seek publicity. This decision was a hard one. We had never needed to advertise; our patients had always found us through word of mouth, which worked because people tend to talk about having fun. I was afraid that publicity would affect the sanctuary nature of our environment, turn our health care professionals into celebrities, and destroy whatever private life we had. Another reason for hesitation was the nature of publicity itself: it's never the truth, it's superficial, it makes us a product, and it trivializes what we're doing by focusing on personalities rather than ideas. However, I must admit that publicity—from magazine and newspaper articles to television appearances to lectures and workshops—probably has been our single most effective fund-raiser.

The first article about Gesundheit Institute appeared in April 1983 in *Prevention* magazine. It brought in more letters than any article thereafter because *Prevention* has such a wide readership. A few months later, an article on the front page of the *Washington Post* Style section also attracted attention when it was syndicated and went to many other major newspapers in the country. Letters arrived by the hundreds. One woman from the District of Columbia telephoned for our address and brought over a check for $5,000. Phone calls came from television and movie producers. Donations, job offers, and speaking engagements poured in. Best of all, enough health care professionals to fill four or five facilities wrote to me, thrilled at the prospect of an environment where they could find fulfillment in service.

Soon after these first articles about Gesundheit Institute appeared, I began giving lectures and workshops about our project and our philosophy of healing. This helped raise money, both for living expenses and for starting to build on the new West Virginia site we had obtained in 1980 (see chapter 10). As I continued to accept invitations to lecture and was asked back for return engagements, it became obvious that many aspects of health care were not being addressed at medical conferences. So I began to add clowning and theatrical presentations to my lectures about medicine. I drew upon the skits we had improvised at home since the mid-1970s, especially those featuring Dr. Niedernamm, a nineteenth-century snake-oil salesman promoting a line of elixirs called "Not-Quite-the-Answer Products." We linked the skits together to make an actual show about the magic elixirs of life: wonder, nutrition, humor, love, faith, nature, exercise, and community. We danced, prayed, flossed our teeth, chanted, and laughed together. This show was an advertisement for wellness and an excellent description of what Gesundheit Institute was all about. We later added a second show featuring eight more magic elixirs: hope, passion, relaxation, family, curiosity, creativity, wisdom, and peace.

Under the umbrella project called "Medicine and Musical Comedy," we received grant support from the Ruth Mott Foundation to produce not only the elixir shows but a variety of other productions that spread the news about holistic lifestyles, community, the joy of caring, the joy of service, and the healing power of humor. We presented humor shows all over the United States, including an evening dance entertainment, a kids' "playshop," and a symbolic skit by Linda and me on the importance of balance in one's life, from physical balance to balance in relationships and in nature. The show featured a gorilla on a unicycle, marionettes, and singing cowhands. We hired ourselves out at conferences, meetings, and parties as lovable, innocent idiots, dubbed "Dang Fools." For one show, I constructed a giant condom from latex, painting layer after layer on a sheet of glass until it was strong enough to lift from the glass and wrap around my entire body. I sealed up the sides and left a hole for my face.

During a visit to Harvard Medical School, I talked for two hours to an audience of medical students from all over Boston. They sat on couches, tables, and the floor and lined the walls of the Vanderbilt Hall common room. Later, my colleagues, J. J. , Eva, Kristin, Mark, Lisa, and I spent half a day teaching sixteen medical students "how to be a nutty doctor." We dressed them in leotards, deelyboppers, angel wings, and rubber noses and introduced them to juggling, clowning, and slack-rope walking in the ivy-bound Harvard Medical School quad.

The response from participants in these workshops was enthusiastic and encouraging. Several weeks after that trip to Boston, I received a letter from one of the "playshop" participants, Paul Cooper:

> . . . the most valuable thing [we] gained was the realization that after medical school we really can do whatever we want and practice the kind of medicine we believe in. . . . Those of us who learned "how to be nutty" saw the universal power of laughter in action as we spread silliness throughout the Longwood Medical Area, bringing smiles to the faces of passers-by, policemen and women, ambulance drivers, food vendors, and, of course, patrons of that fine drinking and TV-watching establishment, the Windsor Bar. Some of the more memorable remarks we heard during our clowning crusade included, "I've been in Boston for three weeks and you guys are the first nice people I've met," and "You guys are gonna be doctors?! That's great!!"

At a preventive medicine symposium at the University of Minnesota in 1986, I later learned that my presentation received the highest marks of all those offered at the two-day convention. The conference coordinator wrote, "Whether any of us end up in a 'Gesundheit' Institute or not, we can all remember just what it is we are about, and learn how to take real care of our patients."

My travels also inspired change. After I gave a "playshop" at DeKalb Medical Center in Decatur, Georgia, in 1989, the Director of Medical Affairs wrote that one doctor surveyed his patients the next day to find out whether they'd rather go to a "goofy" or solemn part of the hospital, and everybody voted for the "goofy ward."

My dedication to goofiness made me somewhat of a media event as my message was spread through radio and television. I appeared on the Oprah Winfrey show along with three other so-called eccentrics. I also participated in a public television program about the Giraffe Project, an organization that gives awards to folks "who stick their necks out." I was one of the featured Giraffes. In 1990, public television in West Virginia produced a beautiful half-hour show about our future facility. For several years I have been negotiating with an independent television producer who wants to make a fictionalized account of the Gesundheit Institute. Some of this exposure might be awful and some might be wonderful, but in either case it will help us build our hospital.

One of my most rewarding experiences, a trip to the Soviet Union in 1985, was undertaken not to publicize our project but to promote world understanding and peace. I was one of seventy-five citizen diplomats—doctors, teachers, artists, religious leaders, TV personalities, movie stars, and even great-grandmothers—who had been invited to reach out to the Russian people in friendship. From the moment I presented the Russian customs officials with my "laugh-port," a humorous passport photo showing me with twenty noses, I spent the next two weeks as a clown. I wore a rubber nose and a funny suit of bright, clashing colors and designs. I had brought a gross of rubber noses and put them on soldiers, old ladies, and kids. Thousands of people laughed as I did silly walks in that garb on subways; in schools, hospitals, and churches; and at formal Soviet peace committee meetings.

Every year since then, I've returned to the former Soviet Union as a clown and met hundreds of people, some of whom are now friends for life. This may be the best thing I do for myself. If any reader is inspired to come, please let me know. Experience is not required. These experiences have made me think that leaders and politicians in our nation and the world over should send in the clowns and put the fool back in court to help balance the intensity of international affairs.

Back when I was in medical school I had sworn never to turn away patients, and when I first started lecturing, I equated fund-raising to doing exactly that. I terribly missed working with patients. Fortunately, my travels and contacts with health care professionals helped ease that loss. In a sense, these people became my "patients" as they participated in my ministering lectures and workshops about burnout and the need for humor and intimacy in medical practice. On the lecture circuit, people thought I was practicing great medicine. Doctors, nurses, and even people not in the health profession would hear about the Gesundheit experiment and start giving service in their communities. So, in a sense, through them I was ministering to the community and society as the patient. But this still did not provide the one-on-one contact that I love in medicine.

In the years since we "went public," I have received tens of thousands of letters from people who want to encourage and help us to whatever degree they can. I have answered every letter. If the letters were piled up, they would probably make four to six stacks, each about five feet high. On a typical day when I'm not traveling, I write twenty to forty letters and conduct thirty or more phone calls, many directed toward building our hospital.

To maintain contact with our growing "nutwork," we started publishing *News From Gesundheit Institute,* later retitled *"Achoo! Service."* Gareth Branwyn and his wife, Pam Bricker, started our newsletter in the early 1980s to keep our friends abreast of our progress, our needs, and most of all our desire to involve them in our project. The first issue announced that we would soon break ground for our first building in West Virginia. Each issue of the *News* reported new milestones toward building our hospital. *News* also tracked our family growth: two home births in the spring of 1987 (Lars, born to Linda and me, and Blake, born a month later to Gareth and Pam); J. J. and Eva Bear's wedding in September 1987; the birth of their baby, the first of our group born on the land in West Virginia; and the purchase of our house at 2630 Robert Walker Place in Arlington, Virginia.

The newsletters repeatedly told of my deep desire to practice medicine again and of my hope that the period of having to turn patients away, which began in May 1983, would be brief. They described the progress we were making on our land in West Virginia and listed the projects planned for the upcoming building season. Each issue of the *News* carried an appeal for funds, and the response made it possible for us to move on to each new stage. Some of the donations were exceedingly generous, but mostly we relied on grass-roots support. Our biggest challenge now is collecting the money for the hospital itself. We cannot begin to build it without a starter fund of at least $2 million in the bank, because we can't build a hospital half way.

In an early newsletter, I wrote of a health care community based on friendship and mutual interdependence, with a staff that lives in the facility with their families in a collective atmosphere of happiness, silliness, love, creativity, and cooperation. This atmosphere will—as it has in the past—enhance health and relieve suffering as no other force can. The practice of medicine will become a joy in such surroundings.

Our dreams about this kind of ideal medical facility have persisted and grown stronger over the years as we have incorporated new ideas. We will continue to welcome new ideas. For the first twelve years, our Gesundheit Institute project was practically unknown, and nobody worked for it except those of us who were seeing patients. Today huge numbers of people know about our dream and want it to happen, but big dreams take a long time to build and to realize.

Whatever happens, I believe that our primary goal is not the creation of a hospital but the larger commitment to having a dream and sticking with it.

PART I

Bringing Vision
and Joy to the
Practice of Medicine

M odern medicine is crying out for hope. The American Medical Association (AMA) and medical and lay writers shout in pain over the direction it has taken. Never have we better understood the mechanisms of body functions. Yet doctors, nurses, hospitals, clinics, and health care professionals are rarely vibrant with the joy of human service. We are seeing a health care system in pain, people in pain, a world in pain. I believe that something can be done to make it better.

In the ideal medical practice, healing becomes a loving, human interchange, not a business transaction. The health care professional reaches out to patients who express their pain and vulnerabilities. This can be the basis for a real bond, even a friendship. Yet, in reality, very few patients or health care professionals feel this closeness. I believe that the loss of this relationship fuels much of the lay criticism of modern medicine, malpractice claims, and the health care professional's tragic loss of joy in practice.

Medicine has shifted from the community level to the corporate level, there to become the nation's number one industry. The care of our population cannot be an industry. How can a couple, family, group, community, nation, or world be strong if everyone's health and welfare isn't a priority? The current focus on business rather than service is causing a lot of distress, both in the cost of medical care and in malpractice suits. That is why, at Gesundheit Institute, we won't charge money, take third-party payments, or carry malpractice insurance.

I have written this book to stimulate hope, collective vision, and community interaction by health care professionals everywhere.

Work toward your ideal medical practice. Find companions with similar dreams or strike out on your own. The joys of medical practice are available to all health care professionals who practice their arts and skills with love and levity. Help one another achieve this joy and wellness.

Lay people also must take part in the design of a new health care system. In every community, it is possible to have a health care facility that operates as a service, not as a business. I know of huge numbers of health care professionals who would leave their current practices to go to a service-oriented model. So, everybody who yearns for a hospital, clinic, or office practice that is fabulous, joyous, and vibrant can make it happen and make it fun! Ultimately, the issue is not only a better health care system but a healthier society.

1 ⋄ A Health Care System in Pain

I believe that health care professionals who feel burned out are not allowing the "enrapture potential" in the doctor-patient relationship.

Burnout. It is the most prevalent symptom of the malaise affecting the medical profession, and the number one topic I am asked to think, talk, give workshops, and write about. Burnout is a state in which people are unfulfilled by their work and are insufficiently rejuvenated. They find themselves giving too much for too long; then something snuffs out the joy and thrill of helping others.

The blight of burnout is so pervasive in the health care system that everyone expects it to happen. Most health care professionals I have met tell me that burnout damages their personal as well as their professional lives. Yet I refuse to believe that burnout is inherent in medical practice. In fact, the practice of medicine can be a thrill—an exchange so fundamentally loving that it's difficult to contain the excitement.

I believe that health care professionals who feel burned out are not allowing the "enrapture potential" in the doctor–patient relationship. Patients unabashedly offer their trust, love, respect, and much more to a physician who projects a caring, joyous demeanor. So why is this joy so hard to come by?

The first cause is poor communication. The joys of relationships are lost if a physician can spend only short periods of time with patients; gone is the thrill of intimacy. If physicians could really delve into their patients' lives and take time to understand the whole person, all-important lifestyle issues could be addressed. Medications are often substitutes for what the patient really needs. Longer visits make physicians' and patients' lives more real, because shared time is a key ingredient in friendship. Without this kind of friendship, "bedside manner" can feel impersonal and superficial.

An imbalance between work and personal time can also foster burnout. Consistently overextending oneself because of perceived responsibility can devastate a person's private life. Belief in indispensability is a surefire path to burnout. Ideally, a healer should practice in an interdependent group of close friends who nurture one another, take breaks when necessary, and collaborate with similar practitioners.

A third cause of burnout is that medicine operates as a business, thereby inviting all the stresses of a business. Patients become customers. Professionals become paid providers, rigid and unable to share the emotions so essential to friendship. Any health care professional who entered medicine to serve humanity is pained every day by its business aspects. Health care is denied to the poor and limited to many others. The relationship to poor patients does not match that given to the well-endowed. Physicians and other healers wear down as their dreams of serving humankind become compromised.

Fear of malpractice suits, another cause of burnout, haunts many health care professionals. Distrust pervades the doctor–patient relationship and wounds it. To guard themselves against legal action, physicians put their patients through procedures and tests that are unnecessary and simply defensive. Anxiety about malpractice suits also breeds blame, which can be a cancer to the team approach so vital in health care, and inhibits intuition, creativity, and scientific investigation. Rigid medical practice becomes mechanical "cookbook" practice. Saddest of all, the malpractice climate denies the physician the right to be imperfect.

Medicine involves a relationship between doctor and patient. The way either of them defines the relationship can drastically affect how the other responds to it. The relationship deepens if the patient knows as much about me, the physician, as I know about him or her. If the relationship is steeped in friendship, love, mutuality, caring, and fun, then the time spent together can evolve into a partnership where each is vulnerable to and trusts the other. This intimacy is the bedrock of a burnout-free practice.

Unencumbered medical practice can allow for a lifetime of building friendships while serving humanity. Healers who feel locked into an unhealthy healing environment need not cheat themselves out of the wonderful exchange of love that can be experienced in the doctor–patient relationship. It takes little time to reach out and hug a patient, to massage his back or her hands or feet in the hospital. Healers, do not be afraid to feel the thrill of helping others. Don't waste a single patient. Try to set aside at least one day a week making house calls and spending lots of time with patients—maybe even playing with them and sharing similar interests.

For my partners and me, the myth of obligatory burnout has been a major impetus for the way Gesundheit Institute has been designed, both physically and spiritually. We want to create a place where people might learn about friendships and family, love and humor, wonder and curiosity. When these major parts of a person's life are restimulated, there is no burnout.

An M.D., R.N., or similar degree confers the freedom to create any kind of healing climate. We should be thankful for the privilege of belonging to such a glorious profession. Thousands of health care professionals want a joyful practice. It's time for us to band together and rediscover the extraordinary, exhilarating treasures of everyday medicine.

The Doctor–Patient Relationship Redefined

The greatest shock I experienced in medical school came during discussions with teachers about the doctor–patient relationship. The overwhelming majority emphasized the importance of professional distance. This meant maintaining a scientist's detachment and dealing with patients as if they were experiments in a laboratory. The "distance ethic" was extended to the wards, where doctors described patients as diseases, lab values, signs, symptoms, or treatments. I was amazed that a group of doctors "on rounds" could hover around the bed of a human being, staring at, poking, and even undressing him or her with little more consideration than was given to dogs in the physiology lab.

Most of the physicians, young and old, seemed more comfortable with the monotony of the IV drip or the wise wagging of the attending physician's lips than with the patient. I often apologized to the patient after the others had left, embarrassed for my colleagues. The teachers who loom largest in my recollections obviously loved and cared for each patient. At the bedside they spoke to the patient directly about his or her life at a level of detail that bewildered many of the students. One student—completely missing the point—said that this "chatter" with patients diverted us from our goals and consumed precious time.

In psychiatry—ironically, the specialty that should deal with matters of the mind and spirit—the need for professional distance was magnified multifold for fear of the dreaded "transference." In group discussions, we students sometimes showed too much vulnerability in front of an attending physician or resident. Whenever we showed any regard for the patient's pain, we were sharply criticized for "getting too involved." And God forbid we should have an impulse to touch a patient! I remember how much positive excitement was generated when some of the staff tried to develop a computer program that could interview the patient, thus eliminating the need for interaction entirely!

None of these conditions improved during my internship; in fact, they grew worse. Under intense time pressures, the human component was confined to simple answers for extremely complex questions. A patient's work history was summed up in a word: what that person did for a living. "Family questions" revealed whether the patient was married and had children, whether the parents or grandparents were living, and what diseases everybody had. That was it. The patient's faith was listed without indicating whether it was an active force in his or her current life. Hobbies, attitudes, and passions—in essence, the "person part" of the patient—were completely ignored. The "doctor-as-technician" tendency seemed to have gone berserk.

As I discovered this cancer within my profession, I started to wonder what it was doing to patients. So I asked them. I heard anger, fear, and despair flow out in a torrent of frustration. Rarely did I see their eyes sparkle for their doctors. If they did light up, it was more often for the physician's professional reputation than for his or her compassion. In a heartbreaking case of lost expectations, I found that doctors and, to a lesser extent, nurses were similarly affected. They seemed to find medicine exhausting, draining, and almost devoid of deep spiritual rewards. And after more than twenty years of searching for one, I still have not found a happy hospital setting.

Medicine, you are blowing it! Transference paranoia and professional distance be damned! Bedside manner has nothing to do with information about the patient! Bedside manner is the unabashed projection of love, humor, empathy, tenderness, and compassion for the patient. Scientific brilliance is an important tool, but it is not the magic inherent in healing. When science tries to keep everyone alive and healthy forever, it fails miserably. The liberal use of psychotropic medications and the custom of resorting to deathbed heroics are just two examples of how science falls embarrassingly, and often tragically, short of its goals.

For the health of the patient, the staff, and the medical profession itself, patients and staff must strive toward friendship in the deepest sense of the word. Friendship is great medicine. It overcomes many of the inadequacies of the healing profession. In friendship lies the potential for both health care professionals and patients to be themselves without fear of being misunderstood. In friendship there are no taboo subjects, and information is not withheld. An imperfect doctor can treat imperfect patients, with forgiveness on both sides. Patients can take comfort in knowing that a friend is in charge of the case. This atmosphere in itself is healing. In the current climate of litigation, wouldn't it be a relief for health care professionals to know when entering a patient's room that here, at least, they are safe?

Doctors should never buy into the lie of professional distance. Medicine is an extremely intense profession. Medical personnel daily see such profound human suffering that "distance" may be another term for repression. But without intimacy how can healers offset the pain and suffering they are so helpless to cure? Physicians need freedom to cry with patients, to hug them and cradle them in their arms, and to receive the same care in return. Human communication without this exchange of love is phony. It is painful to be a fake.

Transference is inevitable. Every human being has some kind of impact on another. Don't we want that in the doctor–patient relationship? Some studies have shown that the doctor's mere presence can

exert a positive impact on the patient's health. The deeper the friendship, the more profound the effect. Often, in my practice, patients
have craved love from some other person (a parent, lover, or friend)
and felt incomplete without it. So I would give them love. And as I
loved them, they too would love me. With this kind of love, a patient
can never say, "I am alone."

I know how devastating loneliness can be. Patients—indeed, all
people—need to know that love is not a matter of control, but of freely
giving and receiving. I realize that hang-ups about sex have encouraged medical personnel to keep a professional distance. Patients will
fall in love with doctors and vice versa no matter how their relationship is structured. These experiences are easier to weather in the
context of friendship and open communication. Some health care
professionals are concerned about dependency on the part of the
patient. But a professional who has been friends with many patients
will have developed the skills to nip adoration in the bud.

Relationships among health care professionals need help as well.
Imagine what might happen if all the people who worked in hospitals
and clinics tried to eliminate the hierarchies of those settings and
chose instead to be friends with the entire team! Imagine having a
staff so fond of one another that simply riding to work or saying
"Hello" in the hall to a coworker is a delight! An upbeat staff can have
dramatic healing effects on patients and healers alike. I believe that
such vibrancy in a hospital would also affect visitors—who traditionally are anxious, depressed, and restrained—in an enlivening way.
This, in turn, would have a wonderful effect on patients. Imagine
ending forever the refrain, "I hate going to the hospital (or the doctor)," and replacing it with "I had a *great* time in the hospital!?

Service: A Forgotten Formula?

It may be the Devil, or it may be the Lord,
But you're gonna to have to serve somebody.

Bob Dylan, "Gotta Serve Sombody"

A lead article in the January 12, 1989, *New England Journal of Medicine*
by a group of physicians proposing a national health program for the
United States began:

Our health care system is failing. It denies access to many in need and is expensive, inefficient, and increasingly bureaucratic. The pressures of cost control, competition and profit threaten the traditional tenets of medical practice. For patients, the misfortune of illness is often amplified by the fear of financial ruin. For physicians, the gratifications of healing often give way to anger and alienation.

Another article in the same issue described a universal health insurance plan designed to solve medical delivery problems in the United States in the 1990s. The same week, the Chief Executive Officer of the American Medical Association (AMA) spoke with great concern for the future of health care delivery.

These major voices in American medicine seem to suggest that solutions lie more in taxes or in universal health insurance than in restructuring the provision of care. They seem to say, "Just give us more money and the crisis will blow over."

In the rising panic, the very foundation of medicine is being forgotten. There is loud rhetoric about medicine as a right, and silence about medicine as a service to society. I believe that the concept of service has become misplaced in the madness of operating medicine as a business. We cannot really reduce the costs, or lessen the sorrows of patients and caregivers, until medicine is removed from the business sector.

We need to return hospitals, medical supply companies, and pharmaceutical firms to the status of servants supported by the community or, in poor communities, by the state. Once deep interdependence exists between community and hospital, the community can create humane ways to care for needy members of society. If all healing systems were shifted to the service sector, competition among health care providers could disappear, and everybody could work together to bring the best possible care at the lowest possible price.

I perceive service as one of the great medicines of life. It is difficult to have a general sense of fulfillment about life unless a person feels he or she has served. This, I believe, is why many women feel more fulfilled than many men: most women have given intensive service through mothering and serving as a lover and friend. Society's highest respect and admiration is granted to those who give of themselves. Mother Teresa, for example, was universally loved. Most good people sustain themselves and their good spirits by their own giving and by following examples that inspire them. Few medications have more power to prevent or dissipate mental illness than regularly giving of oneself. As scientists understand the biochemistry of psychoneuroimmunology better, it will become clear why unabashed service to others has such power to assuage pain and, if not cure illness, at least make it tolerable.

Service is an action word, a perfect antidote to boredom, loneliness, alienation, and fear. Service can impart the gift of inner peace. Service is the physical expression of thanks to the world, an apt way to appreciate the miracle of life. People who give service are free to ask for what they want, knowing they are worth it. Service gives a feeling of genuinely belonging to the human community. Service is probably the greatest call to action by most religious faiths.

So often givers give out, especially when they tackle huge problems like homelessness or our planet's damaged ecology. They too often perceive the effort as a struggle that *must* be draining. Not so! When the environment is supportive and the quest ignites the soul with the thrill and honor of exertion, the person who serves need never feel exhausted again. So let us make medicine a true service. The transition will not be easy or swift, but already there are many people who dare to serve. Join them!

Technology: Friend, Not Master

I won't operate until we have the machine that goes blip.
Monty Python, *The Meaning of Life*

I love technology but not because I'm adept at it. I've never dared to take things apart and put them back together. I know machines only through their on/off buttons. If a machine has more than three knobs, I delegate its operation to somebody else. I'm the type of person Robert Pirsig savagely criticized in *Zen and the Art of Motorcycle Maintenance* for being out of touch with the machine. My friends would like to confiscate my car to protect me, it, and others on the road. And I still love technology and what it can do for me and for others.

The magic of technology in the household has brought comfort, ease, and conservation of effort. The transportation industry has worked miracles for mobility; communications technology has made the planet a global village. I especially love the great inventions we now take for granted, like the printing press, the telephone, the bicycle, and the record player. These and many other gadgets are so much a part of my life that they feel like bodily organs, necessary to sustain life. My love of technology in everyday life is important because it provides security—like a mountain climber's rope—as I contemplate my ambivalence toward technology in the practice of medicine.

Twentieth-century humanity worships at the altar of technology to such a high point that I wonder who is master of whom. Technology has taken such a foothold in our culture that "progress" has become synonymous with "advances in technology." Regrettably, the impact of technology on our ecology and our society has been anything but progressive. Throughout the industrialization of society, the belief that advances in technology are good has been so persistent that little effort has been made to regulate them.

I believe it is imperative that we pay much closer attention to technology—where it is going and what relationship we want to have with it. For every technological advance there have been trade-offs and losses. In medicine, technology has transformed turn-of-the-century humility into modern arrogance. A termite queen becomes such a baby factory that she is unable to do anything else, even walk, and I am afraid that we are producing many doctors today who, in a similar vein, know medicine only as a technological practice. Without their instruments and machines, many physicians feel naked and unable to practice, even though comfort, empathy, and reassurance—so vital to medical practice—require no technology.

When I look at advances in medical technology in a vacuum, without contemplating their impact, I am like a child in awe. Diagnostic machines, like those that produce the CAT scan and MRI, are staggering—right out of science fiction. On a simpler level, just the IVAC machines that administer fluid and drug treatments cause wonderment. They are medical miracles. Once, after attending an obstetrics and gynecology conference lecture on recent advances in laparoscopy, I was informed that much of the surgery of the future will be performed through such a scope. During a break, I toured the exhibit area, overwhelmed by the gadgetry. Later I spoke at a rehabilitation conference and saw the latest in artificial limbs. I held a lightweight synthetic arm that cost $30,000 or more, depending on the options. What made this cost so much? I wondered. How expensive must it become before people will say it costs too much?

The paradox in medicine is that no matter how expensive a treatment or technique becomes, few people will say that it's not worth the cost—if it can even be purchased. What is the value of sight, of sustaining a life? Sight and life, however, are not the real issues. We have reached a point where society says that we want—and feel obligated—to care for the entire population, while in the same breath we admit that we cannot afford to.

Uncontrolled costs encourage greed, which seems to have infected the medical and defense industries to an appalling degree. Perhaps the third-party nature of government funding removes the personal component that fosters accountability. In both these industries, the perceived need is so great, and the advances so impressive, that any financial sacrifice is accepted. Those who champion the other great needs of our society, such as education or ecological management, get a very small slice of this pie because the products are not as tangible or as profit-making.

As long as medicine stays within the business sector, the cost of technology will outdistance normal growth costs because of the-sky's-the-limit philosophy.

I doubt that any company has ever refrained from developing a product simply because it is too expensive for the consumer who needs it. And no matter how humanitarian, the company is unlikely to think the product important enough to donate to society.

In marketing, the goal is to sell the greatest number of devices, no matter how many are really needed. As soon as one machine is purchased, it is likely to become obsolete; the next generation of new and even better machines already is coming off the assembly line.

Meanwhile, residents and students are trained in large, prosperous medical centers with the latest devices, and young doctors often are reluctant to work in hospitals that don't have them. This is most painfully true of foreign residents who, upon completion of their medical training, decide to stay in the West rather than return to their more technologically primitive native countries. In some cases they don't know how to be doctors without these machines. In a related evil, most large cities have far more of these very expensive machines than they need, partly as a lure to doctors and patients. As a result, many of these devices are vastly overused to support their presence. At the patient's level, the cycle is further fed by the constant demand for the "best" treatment, which is equated with the highest technology. This thinking has slowed the progress of other therapies that offer a different form of "best."

Third-Party Embarrassment

I have never liked the term "third-party reimbursement" (TPR). What kind of term is that to express how a society takes care of its citizens' health needs? Who does that mean? What third party? I suppose it means that no one knows the patient except as a computer file. I don't want to put my health and security—or anybody else's—into an impersonal system. Everything I've seen and heard in medicine since 1967 tells me that the TPR companies aren't really concerned about the millions who are on their rolls. They seem more interested in paying out the least amount of coverage and nitpicking to a distressing degree.

Historically, TPR was designed to help people, but more like a distant relative than a neighbor. TPR has become a system designed by businesspeople, and indeed the system has made many people wealthy. Its effect has been to divert medicine from a service to a business. Unquestionably it is the most significant factor in the skyrocketing cost of health care. In medical school the constant refrain was "Don't worry about it; he's insured." We were taught to over-order tests and overdo procedures. It is easier to order tests than provide care or comfort. As a result, the hospital supply companies and medical technology firms have become multibillion dollar moguls of medicine. Yet the health insurers who support these industries act as if they have no role in escalating costs.

If the current health insurance system is failing, many observers say, let's solve the problem with universal health insurance. Don't address the staggering costs, just ask the federal government to pay! But universal health insurance will never cut costs; it will only make them higher. I shudder at the further losses our health care system will suffer if universal insurance becomes law.

What about the paperwork? Today, and under any future universal health insurance system, it remains a demeaning experience for both care givers and receivers. Legions of clerks will continue to be hired for the sole purpose of pushing paper. Reimbursement will continue to be a circus act with many hoops to jump through, often requiring months or even years. I slammed the door on this system as a student in medical school. Once in the emergency room I saw a woman who had survived a car accident that had killed her husband and one child and left her other child barely alive. She was required to fill out forms rather than remain at her child's side!

Traditionally, TPR has been elitist, telling people what kind of healer they can go to and usually ignoring alternative healers. The insured have minimal, if any, input into TPR policies and are informed about rules and rates *after* they have been set. Over the years, TPR providers have increasingly restricted their coverage, apparently for financial reasons.

I also am offended by the cowering that results from society's dependence on TPR. I wonder when the fear of being uninsured really took hold. Patients cower because they see no alternative to this system and are frightened by the consequences of not being covered. The entire medical system cowers because so much of its financial survival depends on TPR. I can attend a meeting of a state hospital association without ever hearing a dialogue about patient care; instead, I am swamped with reimbursement jargon. Often the people attending these meetings sound more like Wall Street traders than professionals dedicated to alleviating human suffering. The bottom line, they seem to say, is found in the ledgers, not in tenderness. This obsession with profit and loss and with coverage for gigantic medical bills hurts the practice of medicine.

We have become so dependent on the TPR system that we seek solutions only within that context. Very little creativity is applied to the problems of health care. The idea of medicine as a service is hardly considered. In the course of a year, I hear hundreds of doctors bemoan the system; yet, few take action to create a new, more humane system based on service.

Several years ago I spoke at a medical conference of an international organization of private physicians called IATROS. These doctors want to preserve the autonomous relationship between patient and physician without government interference. Most participants were from countries with a national health service; they condemned nationalized health insurance severely. Most of what they said about the effect of government interference on the doctor–patient relationship, as well as on the quality of care, was frightening to me. I fear that the United States will eventually turn to that "solution."

TPR is a solution only for an alienated society, which we have become to a critical degree and in which there can be no meaningful healing. The ineffectiveness of our major service organizations—medicine, education, and law—is an embarrassment, considering their great potential for service to humanity. At all levels of society, our alienation from a sense of healthful living has led us to spend far more money on war material, elaborate clothing, cosmetics, and entertainment than on things basic to a healthy society.

However poor or rich, a community must satisfy its health needs. To work toward a healthier society, we must rekindle the spark of belonging that exists in a tribe or community. When a community truly begins to care for its health needs, issues of housing, crime, suicide, drug abuse, and pollution become everybody's problems, and this interdependence becomes the basis for finding solutions. In the long run, the most valuable and viable solution is a grass-roots organization in every defined community that will address and serve local health care needs.

If a health care professional or consumer wants to rekindle lost vigor and imagination, why not tackle problems like TPR, dehumanized care, and skyrocketing costs? The health care system now works so poorly that many sympathetic co-travelers will be found, whatever solutions are devised. We are social beings who need one another. We can no longer afford to underestimate the level of that need.

Malpractice: A Nightmare of Fear

Fear of being sued for malpractice is one of the greatest tragedies of modern medicine. This thief of the joy of medical practice has stolen the physician's humanity. Our society is saying that we don't have the right to make mistakes. Family doctors know that we make mistakes every day, if only by spending too little time with our patients. We must have the right to make mistakes. Medical science is so imperfect that it is impossible to know for certain, before treating a patient, what the outcome will be. Every therapy is experimental, and every thoughtful physician must take risks in attempting to help patients.

Incompetency is another matter: If a health care professional is incompetent, he or she should not be practicing medicine.

The instant a physician carries malpractice insurance, he or she sets up an adversarial relationship with patients and says, in effect, "I don't trust you." Even the most caring, conscientious health care professional enters that relationship in fear and mistrust. *Fear is not the baseline from which to practice medicine.* It prevents many professionals from practicing outside their offices, from offering needed advice, or from trying other therapies. It inhibits intuition, inducing many doctors to prescribe "cookbook" treatments even when they believe them to be inadequate or potentially harmful. There is no room for creativity. Even if a doctor is open to an alternative therapy and considers it a much gentler treatment, fear will often prevail. Over the course of his or her career, this fear leads to exploring avenues of escape, of passing the buck when a treatment does not work. Team care then becomes threatened because one member may be sacrificed as the scapegoat for another's mistake.

Malpractice insurance has drastically increased the cost of health care. Some doctors pay more than $100,000 each year for coverage. Many physicians who want to practice inexpensive, interdisciplinary medicine have had to abandon such dreams or retire early. This system also generates greed. Lawyers hungrily hope that medical mistakes will be made because of the huge fees to be obtained. I've talked with patients who, in the interest of getting the biggest settlement possible, were unwilling to begin a program of self-care before receiving the money from a court judgment. Certainly, malpractice greed has helped transform health care from service to big business.

The entire malpractice system inadvertently reinforces the doctor-as-god concept. If doctors can't make mistakes, they must be perfect. But in the practice of medicine, with all its imperfections, a doctor can expect to make mistakes, to cause harm to patients, and at times even to kill them. We must have the humility to recognize this. Still, I am confident that no one's medical skills were ever improved by a malpractice suit. I would suspect that, more frequently, lawsuits undermine a practitioner's competence.

The "M.D.(eity)" concept also implies that the patient is the passive recipient of treatment and that the physician is responsible for the cure or health of the patient. This is untrue; ultimately, health is each individual's responsibility. Most health problems have major lifestyle components. The doctor is only called in once a certain level of damage has been reached. This is why we will have a sign at Gesundheit that reads: PLEASE LIVE A HEALTHY LIFE— MEDICINE IS AN IMPERFECT SCIENCE.

We must dispel the idea that medicine or science has the answers to all our problems. Science is an inquiry and a process, not a product. No law dictates whether a disease should be handled by a surgeon, an internist, a homeopath, or another type of therapist. The patient and the family must enter into the dialogue of uncertainty and doubt, and voice their concerns. The courage of both the health care professional and the patient to risk grappling with the unknown should be commended, not blocked by fear.

In more than twenty years of trying to find funding for our hospital, few things heat up the discussion like our refusal to carry malpractice insurance. Many people perceive this as our greatest deterrent to success; they call it naive, irresponsible, idealistic, or foolish. They focus on the negative aspects of our vulnerability. From the beginning, we have tried to be doctors who challenge our patients and society to develop healthier relationships. Studies have shown that the least-sued physicians are closest to their patients. In a community that feels like family, one does not punish a physician's honest mistakes.

The primary goals of Gesundheit Institute are to support friendship on the individual level and to build a community on a broader social level. Malpractice insurance mocks these goals. We believe that our stance on malpractice is therapeutic and necessary if we are to build a healthier society. And for us personally, this position is essential if our practice of medicine is to be joyous.

Gesundheit Institute will not carry malpractice insurance because we feel it is unhealthy for a meaningful doctor–patient relationship. We will not prevent individual doctors from carrying such insurance if they wish, but we ourselves will not practice in fear. We want to have many practitioners working together to help find each patient's best road to good health. We want to work with patients throughout our lives together and help them pursue healthy lifestyles so they will seldom need medical intervention. We want to establish such close friendships that lawsuits are out of the question. In short, we want to do our absolute best to care for our patients. I admit this leaves us vulnerable. But the only thing of value we'll own will be our hospital, and we plan to trust and love our patients so much that they will never be a threat to that.

The Bottom Line: Dollars or Health?

It has been said that the American health care system is not healthy, not caring, and not a system. The dollar is the most visible sign of malaise. Medical services are priced at a level no one would tolerate for a minute if those charges were not propped up by health insurance. As of this writing:

•If you are hospitalized, in many states it will cost you or your insurance company more than $700 a day just for room and board.

•If you ever need nursing home care, it will cost you or your family $25,000 to $50,000 or more a year.

•If you need cancer treatment, you probably will pay at least $1,000 a day, with a full course of treatment surpassing the six-figure level.

•If you need a lifesaving bone marrow transplant, it will cost at least $100,000.

• An artificial heart, another modern miracle, will cost at least $200,000.

•Health insurance to cover medical services is so expensive that many businesses are going broke providing it for employees.

• About the year 2000 the trust fund that finances Medicare Part A, which pays hospital expenses, will go broke.

Spending for health care has risen more than any other major form of consumer spending—more than food, housing, transportation, and clothing. In fact, health care spending—yours and the nation's—will more than double by the year 2000, according to the federal Health Care Financing Administration. Health care accounted for 12 percent of the gross national product in 1990 and is expected to rise to 16.4 percent by the year 2000. Two-thirds of this increase will result from inflation and one-third from use of services as the population ages.

Despite these vast allocations of funds, many of the 33 to 37 million Americans with no health insurance go to public hospitals and clinics for free care. But these facilities are cutting back on staff and services. Thousands of public facilities throughout the United States have phased out residency programs for doctors in training. As poor people continue to need emergency room services, burn treatment, trauma treatment, neonatal intensive care, AIDS care, and many other forms of help, they will be turned away.

Americans who lack health insurance—and millions more who are underinsured—know that the health care system doesn't work. They sit in the emergency rooms of public and teaching hospitals, waiting for treatment of ear infections or the flu because they can't afford this routine care at a doctor's office.

The United States spends more for health services than any other nation in the world. The miracles wrought by medical research have never been more plentiful—or less accessible. Partly because of high costs and poor access, the health of Americans—measured in infant mortality rates, drug addiction rates, and death and illness rates for many diseases—is worse than that of citizens of many other industrialized nations.

Our health care system does a terrible job of preventing illness. A large portion of the population is out of shape, overweight, and without assistance in breaking addictions to drugs, alcohol, and cigarettes. A huge segment of the population is bored, lonely, afraid, and in need of help for emotional problems. Sexually transmitted diseases have yet to be brought under control. On the contrary, they are becoming more prevalent—and, in the case of AIDS, more deadly—especially among young people.

One reason we have such a costly health care system is that it offers little if any emphasis on preventive medicine. Relatively little money is spent on preventive medical services, and health insurers give minimal reimbursement for wellness counseling. Hospitals survive and prosper when people are sick; they are not designed to thrive with empty beds when people are healthy.

Overall, there is too little care for one-fourth of this country's people and too much care for everybody else. This leads to misuse and waste. Many patients pay such high health insurance premiums that they feel entitled to a $900 high-tech test for their hearts, when they have no evidence of heart disease, or a CAT scan for their head-aches. Two to four times as many mammography machines have been installed in this country as are needed for screening and diagnostic tests, but only about one-third of women currently get mammograms when they should. Furthermore, paperwork chokes the health care system. Up to 24 cents of every dollar goes toward administrative and billing costs. This practice uses funds that otherwise could provide services for the uninsured.

This malaise is bound to affect health care professionals, both physically and spiritually. America's medical professionals must constantly defend themselves to a public that is unhappy—if not disgusted—with impersonal treatment and an obsession with labora-tory values and dollars. The former editor of the *New England Journal of Medicine*, Dr. Arnold S. Relman, said: "The physicians I talk to are angry, bleak, sullen. Their attitude is bleaker now than at any time in my forty-five years of medicine." Perhaps this is why applications to medical school have dropped 25 percent during the past five years, and why a recent survey shows that most of the nation's primary care doctors are increasingly sick of their jobs. Thirty percent of the surveyed members of this once-thriving specialty say that the health care system should provide *some* form of health care for everybody.

Many health care professionals fear a "meltdown" or collapse of the existing system. The question is no longer *whether* but *how* change should be brought about. Many of the proposed solutions rely heavily on the federal government to bail out the system. Even if this were desirable, it is not possible. The United States govern-ment is too debt-ridden to afford it and is likely to remain so. Be-cause medical services are so grossly overpriced, financing by corporations, small businesses, risk pools, reinsurance mechanisms, rationing, payroll taxes, and catastrophic coverage plans are also unworkable

The bottom line is to control health care costs and the greed that drives them up. Who is to blame? Doctors are an easy target, but what about health insurance companies? hospitals? drug manufacturers? pharmacists? politicians who do nothing to help? lawyers who sue for malpractice? patients who hire them? the rest of us who tolerate and thereby condone this wretched system?

What is needed is a drastic rethinking of the problem. Rather than quick-fixing the failing health care system, we need to create solutions that will excite both patients and caregivers. We must, in a mutual, multidisciplinary effort, tear down what hurts us and heal a profession of healers. We must take medicine out of the business sector and recognize that greed and selfishness have placed society and its health care system in great peril. Our citizens need to feel a sense of belonging and of community. An improved health care system could help to unite society by taking care of all of its members.

Since funds are limited in any society, we must redistribute them to serve the population wisely. People should be able to put more of their money into their own communities, instead of into big, mismanaged government agencies. We must decide whether to buy more bombers or broader health care for our population. We also must decide whether it is wiser to allocate health care funds to greater quantities of transplanted hearts or to cleaned-up ghettos. Personally, I would be willing to forgo much of our military spending and many expensive tools for medical heroics, and funnel those funds into an all-out crusade to reestablish neighborhoods and communities as healthy places in which to live. We must *solve* social problems, not just continue to patch them up.

To make these decisions, we need an in-depth, broad-based forum on how to utilize our money better. This forum might also decide how to regulate technology so that it progresses intelligently yet serves everyone. The goal should not be to have the best houses and latest cars for every citizen, but rather to offer choices at each economic level that ensure a healthy and sustainable free enterprise system. The national goal should be to keep every citizen healthy and medically cared for. The reaping of huge profits from human suffering must stop!

Many creative scientists, engineers, and artists are willing—if asked—to donate goods and services to health care facilities. They would do this not for high salaries but for the challenge of working creatively with others in service to society. The Gesundheit Institute has demonstrated this on a small scale and will continue to do so. More pilot projects, I am certain, would elicit the service of many great minds and hands, proving that large numbers of people are willing to pursue not fame or fortune but integrity in the creation of a healthy society.

At Gesundheit Institute, we are committed to helping other groups create their own ideal medical communities. By our example, we want to encourage others to reflect on and develop an approach to health care delivery that suits the community they serve. Our goal is to be a stimulus, the squeaky wheel that attracts attention and expands the dialogue.

2 · An Ideal Medical Practice

What Kind of Doctor Are You?

Nosey, curious healers who make house calls will have the time of their lives!

Often I am asked, "What kind of doctor are you?" I generally like to say, "I'm a caring, fun doctor." This response catches people off guard because they are really asking "What is your medical specialty?"

Then I explain that my first hope for a patient is to be a friend, to learn and *care* about the patient. I also encourage the patient to be active in creating a healthy life. I try to be open to many perspectives and never give up, at least not when comfort and intimacy are involved.

By this time the discussion is interrupted by the questioner concluding "Oh, you're a psychiatrist!" Actually, I'm a general practitioner who sees the above qualities as fundamental to the family physician. As a family doctor, I treat people as they are born and as they die, and patients who suffer from all manner of physical and mental illness. What I do with the patients may be different, but I deal with the same problems brought to any family doctor: everything from arthritis, influenza, and cancer to stubbed toes, fatigue, and wellness care.

Neither the tools of diagnosis nor the tools of treatment define a family practice. A close look suggests that their frequent use defines for the public a person who practices "real" medicine. These misconceptions arise from the medicine-as-business context. "Real" medicine is paid for by insurance, but there is minimal—if any—reimbursement for relationship-building, comforting, or enjoying time spent with the patient. The conventional tools—drugs, technical diagnostics, and surgery—are the easiest to quantify.

In the current health care system, when a person is sick enough, he or she relies on a residential facility. The focus is on technology-obsessed, hospital-based care rather than on prevention. There is general intolerance of alternative healing methods. Conventional health care tries to conquer death, ignores the community, blames the victim (thereby excusing society), encourages patients to be passive and dependent, and is oblivious to the environment.

A more effective approach to health care, by contrast, would base care in local health centers and programs, use technology as supportive therapy when necessary, focus on prevention, and support both alternative and conventional healing methods. It would accept death when it is inevitable, value quality of life, use community development approaches, protect the "victim," promote self-care, and be environmentally sensitive. This is the model we will follow at Gesundheit Institute.

We will offer the customary throat cultures, X-rays, surgery, and medications, but we will not define our practice in these terms. These are our tools. In today's climate, patients are apt to think that a visit to the doctor is wasted if they do nothing but talk. There is so much overuse of diagnostic equipment, pharmaceuticals, and surgery that people equate them with "doctoring." Thus, it is not uncommon for a doctor to prescribe a medication or order tests just so the patient will think something useful has happened. Businesses reinforce this idea when an employee calls in sick: many refuse to allow a "mental health day" and require the patient to see a doctor in order to receive sick pay.

We are working to build a fully equipped, modern rural community hospital with laboratory services, a pharmacy, an outpatient clinic, and facilities for internal medicine and general surgery. It will also be fully staffed with many medical doctors and other types of healers. In this context, the pharmacy and surgery will become very important, but we will not define the facility in terms of pharmaceutical and surgical services. In fact, holding these in reserve will provide an invaluable safety net while we first try much gentler and cheaper therapies.

We are aware, when dealing with profound illness and death, that tools like surgery are inadequate. But this will never be true of the humble but caring doctor at the patient's bedside. Family doctors choose the tools they feel comfortable with, but they never rely on them exclusively. At our facility we will avail ourselves of all the medical treasures used throughout history, not just the current and conventional healing tools.

Why We Won't Charge Money

Greed is one of society's worst malignancies, and it appears to have metastasized to every corner of the earth. The sense that greed is incurable may well account for its escalation. Certainly one of greed's most devastating symptoms is cynicism. Unless greed and its symptoms are excised, society will perish. We believe that a society must care for its population enough to take care of its needs. Treatment of disease and provision of health care are fundamental to a society's sound survival. These needs should be fulfilled as a gift to its population, not as a commodity to be bought and sold. In a profit-oriented system devoted to grabbing the most income the traffic will bear, the goal will be disease care. In a service-oriented system devoted to keeping the population at its healthiest, the goal will be disease prevention.

The Gesundheit Institute will never charge money for its medical services. If it is to survive, its staff, patients, and friends will cooperate and donate everything needed for it to flourish as a community hospital. We hope to eliminate the factor of debt entirely from the healing interaction. Although this leaves us vulnerable to the wishes of the greater community, paradoxically, we believe that vulnerability is our greatest strength. We believe it is imperative to need the community we serve because the community also needs us. This is basic to interdependence, which we feel is necessary for a healthy society.

We must, as individuals and as a society, stop our worship of things and wealth and put our sense of richness in things everybody can have in abundance without excluding anyone. These riches include faith, fun, and the breathtaking bounty of nature and friendship. Thus, the central focus of our work will be to form very close friendships. Our ideal patient will be one who wants a deep personal friendship for life. By not charging money, we can greatly speed this process. The Gesundheit facility—in which everybody takes part in the cooking, cleaning, gardening, play, and even patient care—must operate as a circle of friends and family, not as a financial transaction.

The closer we become as friends, the more we will tell about our lives and the more honest we will be with one another. We will use love as our most powerful medicine, especially when a patient is dying or dealing with intractible problems and pain. Friendship also enhances the delicate use of humor in medical practice. This kind of medicine cannot be bought or sold. By not charging patients and by having them stay in our home—whether a house or the hospital we hope to build in West Virginia—we are freer to be silly and to build friendships. We also believe that not charging money is very good malpractice insurance.

The creation of powerful community structures whose members feel a sense of belonging cannot occur as a philosophy empty of action. Gesundheit Institute is the result of that action, fueled by community feeling and generosity. We hope that our patients will take the generosity with them when they leave and spread it in their own communities. This is the heart of our social revolution: to take the most expensive service in America and give it away for free.

Alternative Therapies: Room for Everyone

Let's face it: a huge number of patients are out there. Even if every healer of every variety were available, there still would be a tremendous amount of work to go around. Besides, our individual skills are so incomplete that we often need to ask help of other kinds of healers. People are so unique and diseases so multifactoral that we need hundreds of approaches in order to find the right ones and to keep the patient's hope alive. Since there are miracles in all the healing techniques, why can't their proponents work together?

I'm asking for a white flag of peace and an atmosphere in which we can all work together. Competition among healers is not healthy. This is no sport or game. The AMA is not an enemy, and other kinds of healers are not quacks. The AMA is deeply concerned that outside influences are "undermining" the doctor–patient relationship and that its membership is dwindling. With a closed-mindedness uncharacteristic of true scientists, many physicians condemn unconventional therapies without ever taking a closer look at them. Yet if they were to get to know a sincere practitioner of an alternative therapy and speak with his or her patients, I believe many skeptical physicians would see the value of that therapy and perhaps would even refer their own patients.

We must not make our techniques a religion that we follow even when they don't help. We are healers: caring, empathetic, thoughtful friends to our patients. Our magic is not in our tools but in ourselves. If a treatment helps, does it matter why? In *The Illness Narratives*, Arthur Kleinman, a Harvard psychiatrist, has written about allopathic medicine's failure to treat many chronic diseases. He calls for the kinds of care that good, holistic caregivers are trying to offer. On the other hand, surgery and pharmaceuticals *can* be gloriously effective; in their defensiveness, alternative healers sometimes condemn them, echoing the same condemnation they have received from allopaths.

Somewhere in all this conflict is genuine concern that a healer may harm a patient through irresponsible action. But this can happen in any of the healing arts. In the present competitive business context, it is understandable that a healer should claim to use the best system and that the others are less effective or even damaging. The patient becomes the battleground. The issue becomes not the patient's health but the winning of the battle of systems or, worse, the battle for "the market." There are great healers in all phases of health care. If all these systems worked together, a patient's care could be entrusted to an active partnership. This would be beneficial for the allopath, the alternative healer, and the patient.

I have encountered great pain in caring healers who are unable to practice except under an allopathic umbrella. The pain deepens when the unorthodox doctor is taken to court and called a quack. When we find a potential solution to a stubborn medical problem, isn't it part of our Hippocratic oath to pursue it? My heart goes out to all caring health care professionals who have been taken to court for doing their jobs. (I am speaking not of the practitioner who jumps on a treatment bandwagon for economic motives but of the caring healers.) I also am disturbed by the arrogance of the condemning physicians, who seem to me to be reacting out of fear.

We need forgiveness and goodwill ambassadors to draw treaties of reconciliation between opposing camps. Anger and name-calling will only widen the gap. Maybe we could create a place for interdisciplinary care if we shared our joy of exploration of new ideas and therapies, invited skeptics to our homes and offices, offered to use our methods to treat their patients under their observation, gave skeptics scholarships to attend our meetings, and sincerely acknowledged the great values of allopathic medicine.

In bringing about change, underdogs or minorities usually have to prove themselves. Couples in therapy who argue and fight often have a healthy outcome if, however deep the hurt, one reaches to the other across the gap in forgiveness, love, and fun, and says, "Whatever the hurdles, we will be reconciled; however long it takes, we will cherish our togetherness." Maybe if we went to traditional group practices and offered ourselves as partners, bridges would be built. We could go to medical conferences and share ideas. We could reach out to the AMA through a summit meeting where all could come together.

The point is never to give up. Everybody will suffer until we are one healing family. I want no health care professionals to be uncomfortable with my treatments, but I cannot fashion them to please everyone. If we can build mutual respect, it does not matter how long it takes. So often the battle feels like civil warfare, where extreme ideologies do great harm to everybody involved. Can anyone win at the other's expense? I think not.

I believe that arrogance and the economics of competition are at the heart of this problem. One reason Gesundheit Institute has never appeared in court, I feel sure, is that we don't charge for our services. We certainly have experimented with patients in ways that would make many health care professionals cringe, simply because we draw on all the other healing arts. Yet, no legal action has ever been taken against us since we began practicing medicine in the early 1970s, when the climate was even more hostile than it is today. It is important to be cautious in making claims for any therapy. At Gesundheit we will try to respect all kinds of healing and allow all kinds of healers to work together, as long as they charge no fees and open their treatments to observation. Whenever possible, the choice of technique will be made by the patient and family. We will not work toward a single, unifying healing technique. Rather, we will cherish diversity. To work in such an environment is one of my greatest anticipatory thrills.

House Calls: Food for the Soul of a Doctor

In medicine, efficiency means less time spent with patients. Thus, efficiency is a double-edged sword. In the corporate community, great rewards are given for producing the most in the least amount of time. In a business where material goods are the product, there might be a good argument for this. But in a service industry, more does not necessarily mean better. In fact, more may mean *less* of the desired effect. Medicine has tried to maintain its service nature while becoming an efficiency-driven business, but the service part is losing. A product is involved, albeit an abstract one: good health of both the patient and the doctor.

Efficiency puts a greater value on signs, symptoms, physical exams, and tests than on the relationship between patient and doctor. No time is given for nurturing a friendship. An abysmally insignificant amount of time is spent learning about the patient's social history and lifestyle. And most patients know nothing about their doctors. I believe this loss of deep relationship has damaged both parties. The doctor needs the relationship so that proximity to pain and suffering and the inability to cure many patients do not destroy his or her soul. The patient needs the relationship's great power to soothe and heal. I believe that malpractice problems grow from the ashes of that discarded relationship.

The traditional house call was about relationships. Yes, it was inefficient: it took up a lot of time, and who could afford it? But when physicians sacrificed the house call, they threw away one of the treasures of medical practice. It was not just a convenience for the patient, nor was it necessary to discontinue it when medical technology grew too big to be driven around in an automobile. In bygone days, the patient learned about the doctor's home and family because the doctor practiced at home. This was reciprocated during the house call.

House calls are so significant to my practice that I consider a medical history woefully incomplete without one. A person's home is as unique as his or her genetics. It can tell much about that person's disease and even more about his or her state of health. The home is a person's altar to his or her gods—furniture, photos, music, books, hobbies. Indeed, everything that touches an individual has some expression in the home. A look around the kitchen, the medicine cabinet, or living room can tell you as much as—or more than—a blood pressure reading or blood test. It could take days of intensive questioning to learn just a fraction of what a home visit can reveal.

House calls allow doctor and patient to celebrate common interests and explore new ones. Hundreds of times, house calls have opened up new treasures in my life. I once grew close to our mailman and became involved in his health care. Visiting his home was like entering an enchanted forest: he was one of the country's authorities on carnivorous plants. His house was filled with plants—several greenhouses and a suburban backyard with pools filled with all species and subspecies of familiar and unfamiliar carnivorous plants, reminding me of my youthful days in Holland during tulip season. There, in my mailman's yard, the fields were of pitcher plants and Venus flytraps. My son and I were entranced. My mailman had no social life beyond caring for his plants. He spent vacations reseeding habitats on the East Coast. My family even attended a picnic at his house where all the other guests were from the carnivorous plant society.

Relaxing in a person's home and enjoying his or her hospitality creates deeper bonds than can be forged in a doctor's office. The doctor becomes a person to the patient, perhaps even a friend. The house call is so rare today that the patient greatly values the visit, opening up new areas of trust and respect. The physician becomes more caring for patients, more relaxed in their company, more able to ask sensitive questions and confront painful issues. This is the art of medicine. If the patient has a family, the physician meets them, watches them interact, and learns their perspectives. Whatever a patient says about his family and home in a doctor's office will be remarkably modified by what a doctor sees during the home encounter. When a physician plays with the children on the floor, bonds grow stronger. A stay for dinner is a further enhancement of the relationship. With greater intimacy, a doctor may even be able to avert problems or abuses in the home.

I went into medicine to gain this privilege. I went into medicine because I love people. Today's formal medical practice cannot satisfy this passion for me. I *must* make house calls. The house call is a cornerstone of the happiness I have experienced in medical practice. I would like to suggest that doctors who would like to make house calls set aside a day a week, or two afternoons a week, to try it out. Allow extra time and don't charge much—the riches will come back in multiples. Nosey, curious healers who make house calls will have the time of their lives!

Confidentiality: The Only Kind We Want Is Based on Confidence

Under the present system, whatever is said or done between doctor and patient is held as totally private, never to be shared with others. This privacy is considered sacred in the medical profession. But often pain, especially very deep pain, can be relieved if shared, whereas "privacy" may reinforce or enlarge the weight of a secret burden. We humans need one another, fundamentally, for our survival.

At Gesundheit, we want to move toward minimal or no confidentiality in the healing interaction. We feel that this sacred institution is, in fact, a weak link and no foundation for real sharing. We take our cue from the honesty of friendship and from twelve-step programs in which full public disclosure not only strengthens the depth of the relationships between people but also helps to create a sense of support and understanding. If we did not do this in the context of community and friendship, our policy would be destructive; but in the context of Gesundheit, this intimacy has often truly relaxed a pain by spreading it around.

We will, of course, respect the wishes of our patients while communicating our sense that openness can be an important part of a healthy life. This surrendering of privacy is a cornerstone of friendship and an antidote to loneliness. Rarely in our medical experience have people refused this invitation to openness. In fact, many patients have seemed relieved at being able to share themselves with so many, especially in the context of the daily life of our community—child care, maintenance, agriculture, meals, crafts, and play. This practice helps a person act naturally around strangers and quickly feel at home, unlike the experience of a patient in a hospital. Some have complained about the painful consequences of this frankness, but more often than not the complaints have changed with hindsight. The great majority of patients have been thankful for the opportunity to share.

We are all so vast and incomprehensible that we need not disclose deepest confidentialities in order to reveal major "secrets" whose telling could heal us. A lifetime is not enough to explore all that we are willing to share. Some very private people, in fact, disclose legendary amounts without ever perceiving a loss of self.

I once saw Bill Moyers interview Sam Keen, a self-described mystic cowboy, on the subject of personal myth. In Keen's experience, very powerful things happen in his workshops, and also in real life, when two strangers share their respective stories with each other. Great emphasis is placed on the importance of each story. To me, this is the magic of medicine: healer and healee go on a deep personal journey by sharing stories. Our medical experience at Gesundheit has shown that real healing can occur when two people genuinely share themselves. This is why we want friendship as the context for Gesundheit's practice: friendship enhances the disclosure of stories.

Confidentiality makes intimacy much more difficult—a lie, in fact. We are a tribal people who need community. Human beings need a collective that knows and loves their stories. If one has a safe place to practice this kind of honesty, then maybe one can continue it in daily life.

Another very important reason for openness is that it contributes to the maximum safety of all present. Our home and families, guests and patients will be exposed to all who come to Gesundheit. This will include a large number of people who are suffering deeply and who desperately need listening friends. There also will be a small number of disturbed, dangerous people who might want to hurt someone. Their response to our atmosphere of openness and our ability to express our concerns for safety will help protect us. We don't want to be afraid of working with dangerous people. They too need our help.

Confidentiality has sound, firm roots in medicine, providing a large safety net so that patients can entrust their doctors with even the most private matters. Outside of a community context this might be useful, but within a community, confidentiality can create barriers. The overwhelming loneliness of modern society dictates that we try to break this shell of secrecy. We need to join hands and hearts, to value our vulnerabilities, and to surrender ourselves to one another.

Cure Rates: Success Is in the Caring and the Fun

One of the most frequently asked questions about our work is how successful we are. When I explore what these questions mean, the answer invariably refers to cure rates. What a hollow foundation for success, and what a superficial way to look at the doctor–patient relationship! It always makes me think of the ads that say "Three out of four doctors recommend . . . " The cure rate is no more than a guideline for the feasibility of a particular therapeutic course. It rarely mentions the side effects of the cure, the costs, or whether the same results could have been achieved with lifestyle changes. When a patient tells me that Tagamet has cured his ulcer but that he has changed none of his stressful habits, I wonder, "Is this a cure?" In my experience, cure rate statistics usually measure only a fraction of the parameters important to evaluation, over too short a period of time.

If success really depended on cure rates, primary care physicians would suffer great agony over all the patients they cannot cure. This perspective also promotes the idea that the physician cures and the patient is the passive recipient of "cure." Blame abounds when the cure doesn't happen. The doctor may blame the patient, saying the health problem is psychologically induced, or the patient may blame the doctor through a malpractice suit. A doctor who takes total responsibility for curing may be less likely to work with the patient to uncover the root cause of the problem and may be more prone to apply pharmaceutical and surgical "quick fixes." Cure rates can help define the best therapeutic approach, but they can never truly define success.

The greatest successes in medicine involve caring for others. When a patient speaks of the need to be held, do you hold him? If so, that is success. Do you relate to her in the context of her family, friends, community, and world? Do you nurture his or her hopes? Do you have fun? Are you focused enough to *be there* for a patient? Do you feel the thrill that another soul has trusted you enough to share his or her inner, private self? Are you relaxed and free to give honest feedback, however painful? Do you resist being pushed to carry out a therapy you don't really support? Are you humble about your role in helping to cure disease? Do you expose your vulnerability and human self as your patient does?

Have we been successful at Gesundheit Institute? Yes! We have given our time, love, and respect and have felt greatly rewarded at the end of the day. This is the best anybody can give to alleviate suffering and promote healthy living. Since we try to follow our patients for life, and since all patients eventually die, I like to say that we have no cures but are going for the celebrated postponement.

How to Be an Ideal Patient

Without patients, doctors would be out of business. As patients change from passive recipients of paternalistic care into active partners, I often hear them ask, "How can I be a better patient?" I am always thrilled to be with someone who has given thought and action to this question. Just as many patients are dissatisfied with their doctors, I'm dissatisfied with many patients. I don't want them to be passive, dependent, whining, suspicious, or afraid. I certainly don't want patients to think I have all the answers. Instead, I'd like them to feel terrific about our getting together again as old friends.

The first step toward being an ideal patient is to have a genuine, compassionate, loving, and joyous feeling for yourself. The greatest gift you can take to a healing interaction is your own progress toward a multifaceted, healthy lifestyle. As early in your life as possible, choose wellness: celebrate the miracle of life every single day, search within yourself for what you believe unconditionally, develop as many deep friendships as possible, cultivate your sense of play and creativity, exercise regularly, and eat the healthiest foods you can. Often switching to and maintaining healthy living practices will be enough to prevent many illnesses and mitigate those that do occur. Live life so fully that you have no regrets should you become seriously disabled or ill.

In choosing a healer, ask youself what kinds of health care professionals you trust. From among them, choose at least one as your "family doctor." This should be a person you can totally trust with all information about your physical and emotional health. Your family doctor should be willing to explore these areas fully and to comfort you in a manner that is fulfilling to you and your family. Ideally, you should try to find a physician or healer who will also be a friend. Your search should take place when you are well.

If you cannot afford a physician, try to cultivate a helping relationship with someone in the healing arts—a nurse, pastor, counselor, or social worker—so you will not have to pursue your quest for good health alone. This central person should have information about you from all your other healers. It also would be useful for you to have all that information too.

Try to care for your caregivers, no matter how poorly other health care professionals may have treated you in the past. Once you choose a caregiver, enter the relationship full of trust, excitement, openness, and friendliness. There is a lot of pain in the healing arts. Many healers feel burned out, frustrated, angry, and depressed. So act as if you wanted to enrich their day, remind them why they went into medicine in the first place. Try to be relaxed, respectful (not worshipful), and forthright. Seek out health care professionals who love eye contact, touching, and friendship, hopefully through empathy and shared vulnerability. If a healer acts in a way that bothers you, speak up gently but firmly about your concerns.

Be a patient patient. If you hope your health care professional will be attentive and thorough with you, then be empathetic and accept waiting in the waiting room. Medicine is not like fast food where all the needs and solutions are clear and quickly met. Some leisure is important for bonding between patient and doctor. However, if your doctor is consistently late, consider asking him or her to schedule fewer people. Better still, find creative ways to help your healer create a room that is fun to wait in. Offer solutions and even donate your personal time to help create a vibrant waiting room. Maybe it could become an arena for wellness education and healing group interactions. Or it could become a place to try various stress-reducing activities, from biofeedback to meditation. Patients could read books or work on crafts. Or they could use conversations with other patients to soften the pain, open new options, identify resources in the community, exchange recipes, develop new friends, and so much more. At the very least, your offer to help your doctor could deepen the relationship between you.

Please come prepared for interactions with your healer. Examine your life, talk with friends and family, and arrive with as broad an understanding of yourself and your needs as possible. Bring a list of questions and insist on their being answered. Please exclude nothing—and remember, you are worth all this attention.

Don't worry about costs. Get the medical attention you need and pay as much as you can each month. Always ask if there are cheaper alternatives. Shop around if costs are great. Consider bartering your skills. The cost of care has become so outrageously high that you need not feel guilty about indebtedness. The problem is in the health care system, not in your earning power. Consider working as a volunteer for your health care professionals, and maybe even organizing community support around them to lessen their need to charge so much.

Please don't sue your care providers. If you've done your homework, you will be with healers you love and care for. Then you can be sure that they did not commit malpractice. They did the best they could with a very imperfect system. The greatest protection against being injured by the health care system is a high level of attention to wellness.

If you believe in more than one system of health care, then look for caregivers who respect all forms of healing and who respect your decision to use more than one. Ideally, find healers who will work together for you.

By being an ideal patient, you can become part of the solution to our ailing health care system.

3 · Humor and Healing, or Why We're Building a Silly Hospital

People crave laughter as if it were an essential amino acid.

The arrival of a good clown exercises more beneficial influence upon the health of a town than of twenty asses laden with drugs.

> Dr. Thomas Sydenham,
> seventeenth-century physician

Humor is an antidote to all ills. I believe that fun is as important as love. The bottom line, when you ask people what they like about life, is the fun they have, whether it's racing cars, dancing, gardening, golf, or writing books. Philosophically speaking, I'm surprised that anyone is ever serious. Life is such a miracle and it's so good to be alive that I wonder why anybody ever wastes a minute!

Anyone who has picked up a copy of

65

Reader's Digest in the last forty years knows that laughter is the best medicine. In spite of the empirical nature of this truth, the mainstream medical literature hasn't refuted it, as far as I know. The late Norman Cousins wrote eloquently about having laughed himself back to health after suffering from a serious chronic disease. The experience had such an impact that he changed careers late in life to help bring this information to the health care profession. Jokes seemed so important to Sigmund Freud that he wrote a book on the subject. But we don't need professionals to tell us about the magnetism of laughter. With great insight, we call a funny person "the life of the party."

Humor has been strongly promoted as health-giving throughout medical history, from Hippocrates to Sir William Osler. As science became dominant in medicine, subjective therapies like love, faith, and humor took a backseat because of the difficult task of objectively investigating their value. I am astounded that anybody feels the need to prove something so obvious. When individuals and groups are asked what is most important for good health, humor invariably heads the list even over love and faith, which many people feel have failed them. Few people deny that a good sense of humor is essential for a successful marriage. All public speakers recognize that humor is essential in drawing attention to what they are saying.

People crave laughter as if it were an essential amino acid. When the woes of existence beset us, we urgently seek comic relief. The more emotions we invest in a subject, the greater its potential for guffaws. Sex, marriage, prejudice, and politics provide a bottomless well of ideas; yet, humor is often denied in the adult world. Almost universally in the business, religious, medical, and academic worlds, humor is denigrated and even condemned, except in speeches and anecdotes. The stress is on seriousness, with the implication that humor is inappropriate. Health education does little to develop the skills of levity. On the contrary, hospitals are notorious for their somber atmosphere. Although hospital staff members may enjoy camaraderie among themselves, with patients their goal seems to be to fight suffering with suffering. What little humor there is occurs during visiting hours.

The focus on humor in medicine at Gesundheit Institute has often been declared a major deterrent to our getting funds. Still, I insist that humor and fun (which is humor in action) are equal partners with love as key ingredients for a healthy life.

Although humor itself is difficult to evaluate, the response to humor—laughter—can be studied quite readily. Research has shown that laughter increases the secretion of the natural chemicals, catecholamines and endorphins, that make people feel so peppy and good. It also decreases cortisol secretion and lowers the sedimentation rate, which implies a stimulated immune response. Oxygenation of the blood increases, and residual air in the lungs decreases. Heart rate initially speeds up and blood pressure rises; then the arteries relax, causing heart rate and blood pressure to lower. Skin temperature rises as a result of increased peripheral circulation. Thus, laughter appears to have a positive effect on many cardiovascular and respiratory problems. In addition, laughter has superb muscle relaxant qualities. Muscle physiologists have shown that anxiety and muscle relaxation cannot occur at the same time and that the relaxation response after a hearty laugh can last up to forty-five minutes.

Psychologically, humor forms the foundation of good mental health. Certainly the lack of a good sense of humor indicates underlying problems like depression or alienation. Humor is an excellent antidote to stress and an effective social lubricant. Since loving human relationships are so mentally healthy, it behooves one to develop a humorous side.

I have reached the conclusion that humor is vital in healing the problems of individuals, communities, and societies. I have been a street clown for thirty years and have tried to make my own life silly, not as that word is currently used, but in terms of its original meaning. "Silly" originally meant good, happy, blessed, fortunate, kind, and cheerful in many different languages. No other attribute has been more important. Wearing a rubber nose wherever I go has changed my life. Dullness and boredom melt away. Humor has made my life joyous and fun. It can do the same for you. Wearing underwear on the outside of your clothes can turn a tedious trip to the store for a forgotten carton of milk into an amusement park romp. People so unabashedly thank you for entertaining them.

Being funny is a powerful magnet for friendship, life's most important treasure. Nothing attracts or maintains friendship like being a jolly soul. I know that humor has been at the core of preventing burnout in my life. Finally, as a nonviolent person, I feel that humor has often protected me by deflecting potentially violent situations.

In the twelve years we saw patients during the pilot phase of Gesundheit Institute, we had many opportunities to explore the relationship between humor and medicine. Although we greatly appreciated casual humor, it seemed imperative that we deliberately incorporate it into our day-to-day lives to prevent an atmosphere of agony and despair. Some of this humor came from a stream of jokes that patients and staff brought with them. However, jokes die quickly, and we found that for an atmosphere of humor to thrive, we had to *live* funny.

We learned to first develop an air of trust and love, because spontaneous humor can be offensive, and we wanted it to be taken in the spirit of trying. (Cautious people are rarely funny.) It soon became clear that silliness was a potent force in keeping the staff together as friends. And I, as a physician, began to see the potent medicinal effect of humor on diseases of all kinds.

Humor is important, too, for the health of a community, whether a neighborhood, church, club, or circle of friends. It has helped me live communally for more than twenty years. The first twelve years we used our home as a free hospital, surrounded by patients who had great mental and physical suffering. The staff stayed many years without pay or privacy because it was so much fun. As physicians, we also discovered that humor was a major medicine. Humor, maybe even more than love, made our pioneering project work; it would have been impossible without this great social glue.

We live in a troubled world. Many aspects of society are unhealthy or even deadly, and large segments of the population live on the edge. If we are to doctor society we must rely heavily on humor. Often in public a parent and child are at odds, and the frustrated parent is ready to strike out at the child. If I put on my rubber nose and act goofy, most of the time the situation is defused and neither parent nor child has a win/lose feeling.

How can one inject more humor into a medical setting? First, it must be a joint decision by administration and staff. The most important elements of bedside manner are not medical knowledge or skill but the qualities inherent in fun and love. Once the medical establishment has agreed to accept more humor, people at all levels of employment will be willing to take steps in this direction. It is easiest to be funny when people are familiar with one another. Spend time together learning your limits and practicing being funny. Invite patients and visitors to participate. Be open to experimentation and escalate slowly. Expect many experiments to fail and even to cause some pain. Avoid racist and sexist humor. Strive for goofiness and fun, not an infinite string of jokes.

Some hospitals have begun the process already. At Duke University Hospital, humor carts deliver videos, cartoon and humor books, juggling equipment, toys, and games. DeKalb Hospital, near Atlanta, has created a Lively Room for romping. The clowns of the Big Apple Circus in New York City have created Clown Care Units, which visit children's hospitals on a regular basis to bring joy and assist with patient care. The Association of Therapeutic Humor is creating a clearinghouse with information about humor and about people who practice it as therapy. Finally, we at Gesundheit Institute are building the first silly hospital, where the entire context will be geared to fun and play.

There are many avenues to explore. I think hospitals need to give patients a choice between a goofy ward or a "straight," solemn ward. In lectures all over the United States, I ask medical groups which ward they would choose, and more than 90 percent always choose the goofy ward. In any hospital, "fun" rooms could be designated as playful environments for all to enjoy. This could attract many of the community's creative people, forge closer bonds between hospital and community, and diminish the hierarchical nature of current medical practice.

For all levels of staff, I suggest classes, intimate gatherings, picnics, and even slumber parties to cultivate the closeness needed to ensure more humor and joy in the workplace. I suggest creating humor support groups and maybe a place where people come just to laugh. Many hospitals have realized the importance of faith and have included ministers and priests on the staff. The same could be done with humor: hire clowns and playful people. Many large communities have performers and artists who could be invited to bring their specialties to the hospital. Some hospitals might even consider creating space for them, including a well-stocked costume and prop room.

The practice of medicine is hurting at many levels. Patient discontent is so great that many are resorting to lawsuits. Many health care professionals are so dissatisfied that they are quitting or even killing themselves. Few if any happy hospitals exist. Most people *hate* going to a hospital and have traumatic experiences when they do. Yet, it doesn't have to be this way if we make great efforts to change it. Service to people in times of pain and suffering should—and can— bring rich fulfillment. Let us call on humor to lend a hand and make medicine fun.

How to Be a Nutty Doctor

The field of humor in medicine cries out for more investigation. As a guide for ongoing research, I have prepared seven hints for health care professionals. Humor is so individualistic that I suggest trying these ideas in a variety of settings. Remember, *you are trying to make a fool of yourself.* At first this can be discomforting, so log in many hours of practice.

This is not an area to explore if you don't lead with your heart; as with all strong medicines, side effects can be a problem. Your goal is not to hurt people or belittle suffering but to bring fun to those who are suffering. The nature of deep suffering demands some fun as an antidote.

Humor has many faces, and the following ideas represent only a narrow range of possibilities. I emphasize being goofy, so that most of the laughter is at the expense of the giver. Healers who feel this posture does not befit the dignity of their position are absolutely right, but they should remember that dehumanization of their profession has come under heavy fire. If you are concerned with your image, I suggest that while you look for your funny bone, a water-squirting rose would look good on your jacket.

It is time to join laughter with love as major ways to serve humanity through healing. I feel that a lack of humor in faith inhibits many people from following a religious path. People in many Eastern religions follow a journey to enlightenment that requires personal development along an ascending ladder of chakras, or steps. Following this model, we have devised a similar ladder of seven *chuckras* that can help infuse medicine with more humor.

The Masters

A novice—one without inner direction—starting out on a new path should study the masters to see which direction is most suitable. Dead masters abound: Aristophanes, Shakespeare, Molière, and Mark

Twain are just a few choice comics of the past. How sad that so few teachings of the stand-up comedians of antiquity have survived to this day. We of this century, however, are blessed with many film-recorded masters. Go to them for inspiration: Charlie Chaplin, Buster Keaton, W. C. Fields, the Marx Brothers, the Three Stooges, Laurel and Hardy, Abbott and Costello, Lucille Ball, Red Skelton, Jonathan Winters, Sid Caesar, Carol Burnett, Ernie Kovacs, Jerry Lewis, Woody Allen, Lily Tomlin, Monty Python, Pee-Wee Herman, and the entire cast of *Saturday Night Live*.

In God's eyes, surely, most human acts are ludicrous, so I suggest that novices try to find in every situation a cosmic comic tickle. Some great guides have shown that the human condition is laughable even in its agonies. Dante called his descent into hell *The Divine Comedy;* Balzac called the body of his work *The Human Comedy.*

For some people, a few comic mentors will be enough. For others on the nutty path, many teachers will be needed. And don't forget local silliness—look around your community and circle of friends for folks who extract the chortle. Unsung masters abound who can show you the zanydom of your specific locality. Tag along with these characters, and your talents for humor will grow.

Mantras

The mantra for humor is laughter, be it a twitter or a guffaw. There is a great scene in the movie *Mary Poppins* in which Ed Wynn becomes so overcome with laughter that he floats up to the ceiling singing:

> *I love to laugh*
> *Long and loud and clear*
> *I love to laugh*
> *It's getting worse every year.*
> *The more I laugh*
> *The more I'm filled with glee*
> *And the more the glee*
> *The more I'm a merrier me.*

He's laughing the whole time he's singing. Memorize this chorus and burst into song on a regular basis—you'll see how infectious it is. Be indiscriminate in your choice of times and places. To find your laughing voice, experiment with many combinations of the *ha*, the *hee*, and the *ho!* The laugh should not be a silent mantra. The idea is to laugh spontaneously in public at least three times a day for a month. Yes! Gesticulate, modulate, and project many varieties of laugh in every imaginable setting, especially wherever your inner voice says, "Not *here.*" You are standing in line at a checkout counter and . . .

Child's Play

Children are an ideal audience for any pursuer of silliness. First of all, there are lots of them. Second, their taste is indiscriminate; as long as you don't scare them, you'll have them laughing. With all the seriousness that kids have to face and the frustrations parents have in dealing with them, especially in public places, you'll help create a healing community by practicing your nuttiness on them. One of the great bonuses of playing with kids is that it is acceptable behavior in public. So a beginner can become acclimated to funniness without inhibition or fear of censure.

Look to kids for inspiration and guidance in spontaneity, too, for they are funny by nature. Most adults are funny by intent. One of the diagnostic techniques I use to determine whether a kid has become an adult is to learn whether he or she readily responds to humor. Is it any wonder that when freedom of behavior returns to adults late in life, it is called "second childhood"? So practice daily chuckras on children, and at least once a week, go where kids congregate and join in their play for at least an hour.

Assanas

Making an ass of yourself doesn't come easily to everyone, so humorous postures, or assanas, should be practiced daily. For the beginner I will mention only a few facial postures, leaving the complicated body gesticulations for the more advanced. These facial movements should be practiced before a mirror so you can learn their subtleties. Once you have mastered a few, go out in public and try them. Children provide the most encouragement for the beginner.

A warm-up I like is to put on waltz music and have my facial muscles dance to the music. For one facial posture, the Bloater, you puff out your cheeks to their maximum roundness, bug out your eyes, and stare. As a fine ending, pop those cheeks. For another, the

Weirdo, stick your tongue out and off to the side of your mouth, roll your eyes, and make gutteral sounds. These are both great in the checkout line in the grocery store when there's a child in front of you looking over a parent's shoulder.

The wide variety of facial muscles have left this field open-ended for scientific investigation. I advise loonies-in-training to spend half an hour a day in front of a mirror until that short time is not enough. Learn to be comfortable with yourself. The larger the mirror, the better. Wear costumes, go naked, use disguises, but watch yourself and see what makes you laugh. I like to put on music and dance with the muscles of my face and then slowly let the rest of my body join in. When you find something you like, practice and remember it.

Ridiculous Raiment

Here is another area with limitless possibilities. Given the narrowness of fashion standards, wearing anything out of the ordinary makes people laugh. Certainly a clown costume comes to mind for extreme purposes. Take any of your suits and sew on colorful patches—*loud* colors are crucial for giggles. Go to theater yard sales for treasures. Odd socks alone can extract the occasional chortle. I love mixing colors that clash and combining stripes and checks, all surefire chuckle stealers. Hats are one of the easiest ways to have fun. Might I recommend a fire hat or a space helmet with a whirring mouthpiece? My wife once made me a Santa outfit. Who can pull a laugh better than Mr. Ho Ho Ho himself? Try it, say, in March or August. Your patients will love it. Men, this period in history is one of the most boring, fashionwise. Look to history for inspiration, and don't neglect suspenders! I find all sorts of tricks to play with them. The assignment here is to find the worst possible costume you can, and wear it until you forget it's on you. The toughest part is acting in public as if dressing this way is normal.

Props

Here is an area of humor where human imagination shines. With practice, almost anything can be funny. But there are a few essentials for everyone's medical kit. One of my favorite medical supply houses is Al's Magic Shop in Washington, D.C. No kit should be without a laugh box, an instant pick-me-up for any occasion. Oh, how I treasure the things that can fit in my pocket: hand buzzer, whoopie cushion, balloons, yo-yo, or clacking teeth. As you begin to use your props wherever you go, you'll learn the ideal times to use them. No one can ignore the ever-popular lampshade on your head. The key words are these: be experimental. Practice improvising with items that aren't funny: a rock, a shoe, objects that lie around waiting for you to find their ribs. Wherever you are—times spent waiting in line are rich with possibility—take an object and, in rapid succession, interpret it in many different ways. The pet rock industry capitalized on this idea.

A Red Nose

When I was a senior medical student in 1970, I worked for seven months in an evening hippie-style free clinic. It was my first encounter with the depths of human suffering that many doctors see every day. Since I had time to spend with patients, I learned that medications rarely alleviate human suffering. I saw how ill-equipped we are as healers to actually address the patient's quality of life. I saw how this caused many healers to become discouraged and detached. It seemed, upon investigation, that quality of life for patients and healers improved when people medicated themselves with love and laughter.

For a doctor to administer love seemed straightforward, an outgrowth of empathy and caring. But administering humor was something else. I tried jokes, but they didn't have the potency I was looking for. So I chose to investigate being funny. I learned that it's important to be consistently silly so that people will see it's just the way you are.

Working at that free clinic, I pioneered a red nose and then started wearing a firefighter's hat. It immediately brought a light touch to what was often a gloomy waiting room. I wore it everywhere, and that 50-cent nose created many ripples of laughter. Often, while driving in rush-hour traffic, an obviously frustrated driver would look over at me, see the nose, and laugh. I became enamored of the nose.

A few years ago, my mother had her leg amputated because of a lifetime of smoking and poor circulation. As she awoke from anesthesia, my red nose and I loomed over her; I chuckled and said, "Well, I guess you know what it's like to have one foot in the grave!" She laughed, and continued for years to tell the story to others with glee. It could not bring her limb back, but it did spark her hope for continued enjoyment of life.

Nasal Diplomacy: A Funny Path to World Peace

Thus it comes about that, in a world where men are differently affected toward each other, all are at one in their attitude toward these innocents (fools); all seek them out, give them food, keep them warm, embrace them, and give them aid, if occasion rises; and all grant them leave to say and do what they wish with impunity. So true it is that no one wishes to hurt them, that even wild beasts, by a certain internal sense of their innocence, will refrain from doing them harm
                                                    Erasmus, *In Praise of Folly*

The invitation said a group was going to Russia in May 1985 on a mission of citizen diplomacy. Seventy-five doctors, teachers, ministers, movie stars, and other community leaders would meet our counterparts in an attempt to help our governments bridge the gaps between our countries. Surely, I want peace more than anything else I can think of. And it is no secret that I feel our government's diplomacy could use lots of help. But what is a citizen diplomat? The implication was that simply being in Russia, not as a tourist but as a citizen for peace, might have far-reaching results. Could we reduce the "Red Menace" to individuals with families who like to fish, go dancing, feel secure for their future, and be friends with us? So diplomacy took on an air of neighborliness and hospitality. The emphasis was on direct action to improve communication and love between two countries locked in apparent mortal combat. There was no mention of meetings in the Kremlin of the kind reserved for political diplomats. Our mission was to hook up with the Russian people. We even were given instructions to play games like "Subway Roulette," taking subways and buses until hopelessly lost and then enlisting Russians to help us find our way back.

I was thrilled to go. I had visited Russia eleven years earlier with a group of thirteen friends in an old bus that entered the country at Brest on the Polish border. The wonderful time we had there had transformed my sense of "the enemy" into a feeling of great hope. Here was a passionate, generous, dancing population that had been devastated by World War II (20 million Russians died, compared to our 300,000) and seemed to genuinely desire peace. I made friends with whom I continued to correspond. I remember joking on that earlier trip that we were ambassadors for peace. Now we had an opportunity to go with that specific intent.

I could not sow the seeds of peace through conversation because I spoke no Russian. Yet, I didn't want to limit my impact simply to people who spoke good English. So I chose to go as a clown—a fool. I had done street clowning for more than twenty years and knew its power to spread good cheer. The clown is a universal character with a long tradition in Russia. I'd felt, after the previous Russian trip, confident of a positive reception. There is no street theater in Russia. For personal security reasons, citizens keep a very low profile and attract no attention. So it became an automatic ice breaker, a magnet to the curious! And, like the angler fish, once a Russian comes close enough to see the buttons for peace and friendship, next comes the thrust of a warm hand and the twinkling of an eye as a friend is snared. I also knew that children love clowns. If families saw their children loved by a clown and moved to laugh with abandon, our thirty-word peace vocabulary would strike home.

I debated with myself and conferred with friends about the clowning idea. Most advised caution, suggesting that I take the clown suit for special occasions and be "normal" most of the time. There was a concern that the Russians would feel mocked or frightened by someone so visible. I'm often reminded how intense it is for others to tag along with a clown and it was suggested that my fellow diplomats might resent such ostentation. Besides, it's not all that easy to wear a rubber nose sixteen hours a day and maintain a silly walk for two weeks. Dressed as a clown, I knew I'd have to stay in the role the entire time. I suppose it was my past experience that finally convinced me that if I led from my heart, the experience would be breathtaking. Love and laughter seem to be the prime ingredients of peace. I wanted to touch as many lives as possible, show that I cared, and leave a lingering good feeling.

I called myself a nasal diplomat. I made up a "laughport" with silly pictures of me wearing twenty different noses. These would be my official papers if I had any confrontations—so I also had them translated into Russian. I bought a gross of rubber noses. They were my gift of peace to recruit other ambassadors of the beak.

The seventy-five diplomats met outside Helsinki for three days to become acquainted and try to form a cohesive group. We listened to talks on Russian history, customs, and psychology and took a crash course in thirty words of peace and friendship. I dressed and acted the clown to help folks get used to my foolishness. When I first arrived, I sensed that a fair number of my colleagues were disconcerted by my plan and even thought it was out of place on such a serious mission. However, by the end of the orientation, I received much positive feedback about helping people relax and be themselves. For many, entering the totalitarianism of the country was anxiety-producing. I gave a mini-workshop to my fellow diplomats called "How to Be Nutty" and presented each with a rubber nose to use at will.

Before we entered Russia, several previews of nasal diplomacy occurred. One evening in the lounge of the hotel, Linda and I sat near a dozen Finnish men who were celebrating after a day-long seminar for bank employees. We were enjoying one another's company when one asked why I was dressed as a clown. This led to several hours of uproarious laughter, singing, and sharing of cultures as we were assimilated into their celebration with hugs and best wishes.

Then we entered Russia. We were scheduled to spend eleven days in Leningrad and Moscow. The experience exceeded my wildest dreams. Everywhere we went, people of all ages laughed spontaneously and saluted in friendship. Formal situations were often transformed into more relaxed occasions. A recurrent, refreshing impression, which continued for the whole eleven days, was the unguarded, spontaneous, beaming smile. When we drove into Leningrad early the first morning and passed people on buses and street corners, I saw my happiness reflected in their faces. What magic! Our first stop was a large square at the Winter Palace among a fleet of tourist buses, mostly filled with Russians visiting the site of their great revolution. I approached groups with my funny face and silent joy—enthusiastically shaking hands and hugging—and received many invitations to pose in their group pictures, amid muffled twitters and giggles. On my colorful clownish raiment were buttons calling for peace between our nations. These brought enthusiastic expressions of goodwill. These meetings often ended in tearful hugs and chants of *mir i druzhba* (peace and friendship). For dessert, out came the family photos, and the soulful meltdown of barriers was complete. I'm speaking not of a few isolated thrills but of a scene that repeated itself wherever we went.

One day a handsome man, dressed Ivy League style, stopped me and said in perfect English that he had been watching me, liked my interactions with the people, and wanted to get together. Thus, nasal diplomacy gave Linda and me what became our most intimate and lasting friendship of the trip. We spent every day in Leningrad with Alex and his girlfriend, Sveta. He skipped work and followed us to Moscow. Alex was 30, a graduate student of English, and a librarian and part-time guide and translator for the Hermitage Museum. Sveta was an architecture student. What perfect hosts! Alex was a true lover of all things American; he had just received an order from an L. L. Bean catalog. Conversation never stopped, and we explored all subjects. I was amazed by his grasp of slang, which he beamed at us in a steady stream.

Alex and Sveta took us to many nontourist restaurants that had dance floors. How the Russians love dancing! The band played everything from folk to Michael Jackson. People of all ages danced singly, in mixed couples, and with others of the same sex. To our delight, the Russians readily approached others' tables to ask some- one to dance, even a member of a couple. We had many offers to give celebratory toasts, and one table sent a love letter. We went back to Alex's home because he was anxious to see a John Denver special on TV. During those five days we ate in a pizza parlor (a big hit in Russia in recent years), saw a Las Vegas review show, visited the Dostoyevsky house, and took a romantic row on a network of canals in a park near Alex's home. Our last moments together in Moscow were at 3 A.M. in Red Square, where Alex and I were the only two people—singing songs, laughing, and planning our future. We parted knowing we would meet again and have exchanged many letters since.

Another touching moment occurred in Leningrad. Three of us were walking on the street, absorbed in thought, when suddenly I felt a soft, tiny hand in mine. Looking down, I found it belonged to a four-year-old girl, walking with her father, who had seen a clown and simply wanted to hold his hand. We exchanged love and noses and moved on joyously.

I've always been fond of teenagers, and Russian teens were a ready audience. From a block away, I would spot groups of them returning from school. They would see me and burst out laughing, which was my cue to approach them and enhance their giggling machines. I would put my arms around them and walk with them, never feeling any tension or resistance. I might hold a hand for half a block while we spoke of peace. These teens projected an air of innocence reminiscent of the United States in the 1950s. In a dramatic shift since our trip eleven years earlier, the Russians wore much more colorful clothing and expressed themselves more on the street. One young girl came up to me outside a museum, pinned a button of her province on my jacket, and blushed.

One day in Red Square, I was with two musician friends from the trip. In good weather, the huge square is a festive place, filled with all manner of tourists. Many groups had come from all over Russia to celebrate the fortieth anniversary of their victory in World War II. We paused to watch a large group of men and women, chests covered with medals, posing for a photo. They obviously were country folk, awkward in their drab, seldom-used suits, celebrating in this city of nine million. We began playing Russian folk music, and I danced with an older woman while the others cheered and clapped. This kicked off a long period of button exchanges, photo taking, and chants of peace and friendship. The Russian people we met seemed very quick to reach for any banner of peace. I never encountered any anti-American feelings. It was hard to end that Red Square experience; I felt that as long as it lasted, war could never come.

One final experience came at the Moscow Circus when our lovely guide, Helen, arranged for me to meet the clown at intermission. It was a dream come true. I was laden with gifts of jazz cassettes, a rubber nose, homemade juggling balls, and an offer to return someday to do some street clowning in a combined United States–Russian effort. The clown invited me to return after the show and meet his family. He surprised and delighted me by giving me his beautiful, handcrafted kid-leather clown shoes, saying, "I've made people laugh here wearing these shoes for twenty years. Now it is time for you to do the same at your home." He said he too hoped that through humor the world might grow closer in peace.

I have continued these clown trips to Russia every year since 1985, and each time the impact is greater. The last four trips have each been limited to twenty participants who agree to come as clowns. We range in age from twenty to seventy-eight. We go to hospitals, orphanages, and prisons, and we put on street theater. In 1991, some Russians joined our trip for the whole period; now they are forming a Moscow Clown Alley.

Years after this experience, I remain committed to diplomacy in everyday life. I knew clowning promoted peace but had never done it for two weeks in a row. I now recognize that one need not leave home to practice diplomacy. I find myself wearing rubber noses more than ever, enjoying their tension-releasing power. There are many tools of diplomacy, and I hope that everybody can find suitable ones. If each of us were to use these tools locally to bring peace to friends and neighbors, we surely would have a beneficial effect on the world.

And what a serious world it is! Newspapers, TV, and other media project a huge burden of problems. What if the fool were reinstated at court? When I picture a Geneva talk, I picture international negotiations—what if each head-of-state brought his or her favorite silly person for balance? I believe it would ease tensions and encourage vulnerability for the common good. Lighten up, world! Consider a career in nasal diplomacy!

Fun Death

Death has had a lot of bad press. Many living hours are spent in dread of this great mystery. Dying is one of the few things everybody must do, but often we cannot bear to think about it. Our society is so uncomfortable with death that despite the incredible concern about it, few people are willing to discuss it openly as a stimulating topic of conversation.

If death is mentioned at all, it is usually in whispers—even secretive tones. Is this "deathism"? Does something about our upbringing, reinforced by our education, the arts, and even the medical profession, perpetuate the myth that death is not part of nature's great design but some horrible trick or punishment? Must we buy into this Grim Reaper routine? Are we not free to choose how we look at death?

During my medical training, no one ever gave us a lecture on death. This is a terrible oversight. People die. Lives are shattered by the fear of it, and families are devastated when it occurs. Yet medical education ignores it. The implication seems to be that death represents a therapeutic failure. This is an insidious trap for a physician, who should approach medicine with far more humility. Physicians are not here to prevent death! We are here to help patients live the highest quality of life and, when that is no longer possible, to facilitate the highest quality of death.

If we physicians cannot be fully comfortable with death, we are cheating ourselves and our patients out of a glorious swan song. When I began to practice ward medicine during my third year of medical school, it became obvious that death was the most discomforting fact of life. So often patients who were obviously dying were neglected: left to die. "There is nothing we can do," the staff said. The only time physicians seemed comfortable with a dying person was during a Code Blue, when state-of-the-art medicine was aggressively applied. If the attempt was unsuccessful, everybody felt they had done their best—which, of course, they had. But it appeared to me that for many professionals, this resuscitation attempt was an exhilarating final heroic effort to save the patient. I believe that dealing with dying is where the art of medicine begins. It is a fault of modern medicine that physicians cannot see the potential to make the last rite of passage a wondrous experience.

There is no greater validation of faith than the fact of death. There is no greater reason to develop a belief system and surrender to it. Whether one's belief system suggests nothingness or immortality, either can ease the act of dying.

It is important for a physician to explore a person's faith and perspective on death as a routine part of the medical history. If these views are not clearly defined, part of the treatment should be to define them. I find most patients grateful for the time spent on these matters, and it bonds our relationship. Whenever I spend time with a dying person I have, in fact, found a living person. The young who are dying have been most vocal about this. I remember an eleven-year-old girl who had a huge bony tumor of the face with one eye floating out in the mass. Most people found it difficult to be with her because of her appearance. Her pain was not in her dying but in the loneliness of being a person others could not bear to see. She and I played, joked, and enjoyed her life away. This is when I made a commitment to enjoy the profoundly ill and act normal around them.

Another friend in his early twenties with cancer said emphatically that he was a living person and hated the discomfort people showed about his dying. That discomfort, he said, interfered with his life. He went to a big dance shortly before he died and, with only part of one lung left, danced longer and harder than most of the people present. *Dying is that process a few minutes before death when the brain is deprived of oxygen; everything else is living.*

When I began medical practice, I had to decide how I was going to address the issue of death. I took my cue from nineteenth-century literature. Novel after novel described home death experiences that were wonderful for both patient and family. It made great sense. What could possibly be better than to die in the company of family and friends, surrounded by home and treasures one had lived with? In the hospital, dying people I interviewed felt lonely and estranged from their environment. What perked them up were visitors and a few mementos of their lives that were kept nearby. When I spoke to health care professionals, few if any felt this was how they wanted to die. Many said that when their time came, they would end their lives with medication.

So I encouraged patients to die at home and agreed to attend to them there. Each time I have done so, a great deal of fear has been removed from the death experience. Each time, patients and family have been deeply grateful, often experiencing the same joy and exhilaration as at a home birth. These families are among the most thankful I have known. I realize how few people today have ever fully experienced the death of a loved one. When I was sixteen my own father died in a hospital with no family around and no chance to say good-bye. I feel angry and cheated that I was not with him.

Consider the parallels between birth and death. For most of this century, birth in this country was a painful experience, with the mother sedated and the father and family kept at a distance. When I was in medical school, the obstetrics rotation was in a city hospital with thousands of births a year. Women screamed in pain for hours, tormented by the hospital routine and needing sedation. Doctors behaved as if *they* brought babies into the world, whereas in truth, women are the ones who give birth! Very early in my practice, I attended home births and had a completely different experience. Here was a celebration of the highest order that bonded the entire family, with the midwife or doctor simply serving as a guide.

If birthing classes can make birth a glorious experience, why not have deathing classes to prepare us for death? Often, making a life experience familiar has eased anxiety about it. That is why I advocate fun death. I have asked thousands of people how they feel about their deaths, and I hear these recurrent themes: "I don't want it to be painful" and "I want it to happen in my sleep." I believe that with conscious effort and advance planning, dying can be an anticipated and beautiful event shared with one's family and friends—a final celebration of being together.

So I ask patients to imagine what kind of death they would want. "What would be your ideal?" I ask. "Do you want a miserable, anxious death, alone in a hospital, with everybody acting as if you're already dead? Or would a fun death be more to your liking?" By "fun," I simply mean whatever that individual considers ideal, within the limits of feasiblity.

At our proposed hospital, and in the homes of patients who wish it, we will involve terminally ill patients in planning their deaths. We will encourage dialogue with their families so the patient's wishes are clear to all. In suggesting a fun death, I hope that patients and their friends will use their creativity to design a death experience that is not only comfortable but downright anticipated. Because we will have a willing staff and many props, I'd like to think that whatever is desired will be acceptable, as long as patients have made their wishes clear to their families beforehand.

Some might prefer a quiet death at home with family and clergy gathered in prayer, welcoming the coming of eternity. Some might prefer three women in black, crouched in the corner moaning. Others might ask their friends to dress as angels, playing harps and singing of coming attractions. A wild dance party might suit some. For myself, since I'm a silly person, I would like a silly death. The key is personal choice.

In no way am I trying to ignore or belittle the tragic loss of the deceased to the family and the world. We all must experience that loss and grieve in our own style. This exercise is intended for the dying person, not particularly for those still living. That is why it is so important for patients to communicate with their families. Most patients I've spoken with want only to be home with their loved ones and in familiar surroundings, perhaps with some music, massages, prayers, and memories added.

Contemporary society is experiencing a major breakdown of family structure. It's time to glue it back together again. The intimacy of planning and creating an intimate death experience would form that kind of cement. Let's stop fearing death and transform it into an experience that could bring us closer together as a family. Let's have a fun death.

4 • Art, Nature, and Imagination

Art, nature, and imagination are fundamental to health care. They are not expensive embellishments to a scientific practice. I consider them essential to maintaining wellness and caring for disease. So much healing goes on through their influence—on both caregiver and patient—that it is important to include these great medicines at the core of our medical work. Involving them makes it possible for a doctor to respond intuitively to a patient's problems and ensures sensitive treatment, not a textbook solution.

Nature tops the list of potent tranquilizers and stress reducers. The mere sound of moving water has been shown to lower blood pressure.

Art as Primary Care

As a primary care family doctor, I consider the artist a peer, and art is as much my stethoscope as my scalpel: necessary for both diagnosis and treatment. This has always been so. I cannot conceive of practicing medicine without art, either in my life or in my patients' lives. In Gesundheit Institute's dream hospital, every square foot of space devoted to the arts is as essential to diagnosis and treatment as the surgical suite or hydro-therapy room. Art is not an indulgence, secondary to medical activi-ties, but is fundamental to the practice of interdisciplinary medicine.

The words *art* and *medicine* have long been associated. The mean-ing of "science of medicine" is quite clear and includes technology, pharmacy, and research. But what does "art of medicine" mean? Art is the style in which science is employed, a bedside manner, the way one conveys compassion, promotes staff harmony, or communicates. Art's action verb, create, includes ways of seeking solutions, pursuing research, and balancing complexities. Creativity is the process of making or bringing into being. So a creative act, such as providing high-quality care, is a product of one's artistic self. Thus, one can find art in walking through a ward or in drawing blood.

This leads to the use of art in promoting wellness and preventing disease. Creativity is great medicine for the creator, and the end result can be great medicine for whoever experiences it. I am sure that if creativity were ever studied, it would prove to be a great stimulant for the psychoneuroimmunological core of each individual. Creating things together bonds people and stimulates deep, intimate conversa-tion. In our hospital, staff members will be encouraged to follow all their artistic interests and to include patients and guests. This will go a long way toward preventing burnout and enhancing relationships. Guests and patients will be encouraged to follow their interests, teach others, and provide for the facilities' pleasure and environment. This way, they can feel they are giving to the community, not just taking.

Our art "umbrella" will include literature, visual arts, performing arts, crafts, architecture, philosophy, and religion. Already they are in use as art therapy, psychodrama, music therapy, dance therapy, and puppet therapy. But I want to avoid letting these narrow definitions confine how these activities may be used in the healing arts. Our community held regular dances for years, during which I learned much about people: how fit they were, how tense, how creative. One can observe gender boundaries and mating dances. The celebration around a dance is a great social grease and a fine way to enhance communication, relationship, and a sense of belonging. One fascinat-ing thing I learned was that when many people danced, any one person was physically able to dance much longer than when only a few danced. It was a dramatic expression of exchanged energy. I often used art books to help draw a patient out, by trying to think which artist in history might trigger important growth or interaction. Whenever we made a movie or produced a play, the discussion and fun enhanced the medical practice. I am as thrilled that our hospital will have a modern stage as I am that it will have an emergency room. In either case, we will be prepared to handle whatever comes to us. The many plays dealing with AIDS, for example, demonstrate how art helps us address health and social issues.

Art has great power to uplift, communicate, enhance understanding, educate, and impart beauty. Art always has facilitated gentle social change. To this end, artists from all over the world have donated, and will continue to donate, work to grace our walls, gardens, and other spaces wherever a piece, by its presence, may change lives. Our favorite cartoonist has agreed to create goofy murals in keeping with the comic flavor we want. Because we believe that beauty heals, our architecture and landscaping will have an esthetic that soothes and stimulates. We recognize that our constructed environment has a strong impact and cannot be taken casually or allowed simply to provide the function of space. There will be countless ways of stimulating all the senses at Gesundheit.

Creativity and play will be cornerstones of our ability to keep old staff and attract new. Art always has played a role in social organization. Creativity and play likewise will be important tools to emphasize our messages of wellness, service to humankind and nature, and relief of suffering. Art and its countless expressions are more than important adjuncts to medicine; they are the heart of its successful practice.

Nature, Justly Called Mother

> *Earth fills her lap with pleasures of her own;*
> *Yearnings she hath in her own natural kind;*
> *And, even with something of a mother's mind,*
> *And no unworthy aim,*
> *The homely nurse doth all she can*
> *To make her foster-child, her inmate Man,*
> *Forget the glories he hath known,*
> *And that imperial palace whence he came.*
> William Wordsworth, "Ode: Intimations
> of Immortality from Recollections of Early Childhood"

It is with profound wisdom that the words *Nature* and *Mother* are wed. Mother symbolizes comfort, someone to seek whenever one is troubled. The potential always is there to be comforted and forgiven, for nature is omnipresent. Inherent in becoming nature's offspring is the glorious opportunity to live with a feeling of belonging. For this reason alone, it is important to integrate nature with healing work, to give Mother Nature room to contribute to relaxation and stress reduction. A simple blade of grass or a spectacular vista, an untouched wilderness or a meticulously planned garden, can hold any person transfixed. A lifetime is not enough to explore a fraction of nature's breadth.

Many people, young and old, have never made the nature connection or have lost it along life's way. Today's children stay indoors so much that many of them never have an opportunity to discover the treasures beyond their front doors. Getting lost in the woods is more frightening than adventuresome. Obsessions with cleanliness create phobias about dirt, bugs, and getting wet. Modern multimedia stimulation has usurped the simple pleasures of bird-watching or going for a walk. Nature can easily match or surpass our technical pleasures but doesn't have enough advocates supporting that ethic. There has been such a chasm between humans and nature that the connectedness is largely ignored. A dominant arrogant philosophy even says that nature exists to serve *us*. This has led us to perpetrate such tremendous abuses on nature that we have reached the point of a potential environmental holocaust.

We must resume our place as one of the life cycle's many players and stop being part of the problem. The core of a wellness/prevention lifestyle must include prevention of ecological disasters like deforestation, aquifer depletion, desertification, loss of topsoil, air pollution, water pollution, and the extinction of many species of animals and plants. To this end, Gesundheit Institute will emphasize nature issues as zealously as it does health issues. At our site in West Virginia, the creek, wet and dry bottomland, four-acre lake, waterfalls, forested mountain, natural caves, acres of ornamental and herb gardens, and wide variety of walks, paths, and stopping places will allow nature full expression in all seasons. Patients and staff will learn conservation formally through lectures and informally through play and working together on the land. They will learn to draw parallels between life and death in nature as well as in themselves. Experiments in appropriate technology, agriculture, and landscaping will reveal healthier ways to harmonize humans and nature. We will support other such experiments and will explore healthier ways to recycle and deal with waste.

For a personal sense of wellness, we will use nature to eliminate boredom by rekindling wonder and curiosity. Whether walking up our mountain, fishing in the lake, or studying with a microscope, patients and staff will find rapture in nature's bosom. Nature also teaches humility: grandly through earthquakes and floods and subtly through weather and plant blight. It is important for humans to feel their fragile vulnerability and reduce unhealthy arrogance.

Nature, the attending physician, will help us explore beauty and inspiration. The gardens will have a palette of color, sound, smell, and touch that will melt even the hardest heart. Everybody will have a hand in creating the gardens. To augment our messages about good nutrition, patients will help plant, tend, harvest, preserve, and prepare food, and thereby take more interest in what they eat and where these foods come from.

Among nature's therapeutic values is her ability to heal mental illness and anguish as few other forces can. Often I have gone outside with a psychotic person and hugged a tree for a long time or rolled down a hill. Nature tops the list of potent tranquilizers and stress reducers. The mere sound of moving water has been shown to lower blood pressure. Nature, I have found, is a key medicine for the profoundly ill and dying when all else has failed. Nature is so useful in building a therapeutic relationship between patient and health care provider that an hour's walk together in the woods can have far greater impact than an hour spent on either side of an oak desk.

Gesundheit will be an ideal place to find "power spots": special places for people to go to examine themselves, make important decisions, and relax. Those who feel uncertain about their lives will find opportunities to go on a vision quest to find a healthy direction to take. We will send a dozen or so people on seven-to ten-day hikes in the wilderness. They will ford rivers, make camp, cook meals, and experience human bonding, cooperation, self-care, fun, and much more—all thanks to nature.

Finally, I'd like to point out that humans *are* a part of nature. People who love the country and dislike the city often extoll nature's abundance as if it existed only in the country. I love the city *because* of its nature—because of *people!* Crowded malls are as heavenly to me as a forest; all those people are trees to me. Gesundheit brings people together and teaches them to love their quantity as well as their individual qualities. If we humans don't learn the former, our survival is in question. Inside Gesundheit's walls, we will be a small-scale human mall and nature will be us. Outside, we will enjoy the rest of the natural world as we find ways to work and play with all its many forms.

Imagination

No universe is more vast than the imagination. Everything passes through it first: all arts, philosophies, and inventions, to name a few, and every modification and sidetrack as well. Imagination is the best friend of the conscious mind, the dream tinkerer, and life's happy companion. Throughout history, we have often stopped external activities (or made them repetitious) in order to enter the infinite regions of the mind, from casual daydreams to disciplined meditations.

Endless, boundless, colossal—we cannot confine imagination to adjectives alone because even in our choice of description, imagination is in control. It defines itself. Cerebral spontaneity pulses into being like a birth. Thought, the foster parent, takes its child and acts— or doesn't act—as it sees fit. Where does imagination come from? Thought can provide only the crudest steering mechanism. The rest is an eclectic ocean of collective conscious and unconscious memory. All that is a person's history and every possible permutation and combination of sensual input begins as imagination's seed. Three thousand million years of computer design could not begin to contain or simulate imagination. I suspect that in another thousand years, science may begin to dissect imagination's biochemistry. Meanwhile, I prefer to think of imagination as a marionette with a million strings. All we see is the final product: our next moment of imagination.

All the cultures that ever existed, with every one of their achievements, represent only the broad strokes of imagination's handiwork. Every single issue (and every permutation of every issue) of life is toyed with inside the imagination. Where is this more evident than when we fall in love? The poems and songs inspired by the love-bent imagination dominate the history of spoken arts. Love is one of imagination's intoxicants.

For many people, imagination peaks between the ages of two and five. After that, its use declines and boredom rises. Many people put their imaginations to sleep rather than eliminate them altogether. Boredom is an insult to the miracle of life and an abandonment of thankfulness; it is at the heart of human suffering. Few forces have more power to heal boredom than playful imagination. As a physician, I consider it a medical emergency if I perceive that an adult has allowed imagination to flounder and boredom to take hold. Boredom can be eliminated simply by nourishing the imagination. People who say "I have no imagination" project the body language of being dead. Everything comes from the imagination: its sacred graces can make life sparkle and make a person young at heart.

Everybody can stimulate imagination; it exists in every person. Like the physical body, imagination can become flabby if it is not exercised and appreciated. Here are some qualities that exercise the imagination:

- A glorious sense of wonder through contemplation and study of nature, humanity, the arts, and life itself

- Curiosity about everything and everyone

- Exploration of all areas of interest, however briefly, and saying yes to every opportunity

- Sharing of ideas with every available person and studying ideas very different from one's own

- Enormous sense of play and improvisation, with huge quantities of goal-free experimentation

- Tinkering in every artistic medium

- Restructuring of thought; time away from rehashing problems, worry, fear, and doubt; imagination gymnastics, such as picturing a world where chlorophyll is some color other than green . . . maybe thirty different shades

- Restructuring one's life toward happiness

Bringing imagination into medical practice makes a physician not only a better doctor but a better human being. What stronger basis can there be for the practice of medicine?

5 · Rebuilding Self, Family, Community, World

I graduated from medical school "head smart." While living in community, however, I have built buildings, farmed, raised goats, produced movies, and learned rope walking and unicycling.

The most distressing health problem for many people is the combination of boredom, fear, and loneliness. Our health is damaged most by loneliness and lovelessness. If relationships with our families, friends, and ourselves are not going well, no amount of physical health can compensate. Huge numbers of physically healthy people lead miserable lives. Conversely, if our relationships to family, friends, and self are strong and sustaining, then even a dying person can enjoy the bliss of community.

The parallel in medicine is the relationship between healer and patient. During the years that we actively saw patients at Gesundheit Institute, everything we did, as individuals and as a community, was directed toward building intimacy and friendship. If someone came over to work in our garden or enjoy one of our theatrical productions, that helped build a healing relationship. Such activities were healing in an even more profound sense because loving a person and making that person a friend foster self-esteem. Some people may take twenty years to develop such a friendship. With others it happens rather quickly. Playing together, talking and listening to one another, doing projects together—all build self-esteem.

But intimacy and friendship are not a part of conventional medicine. There the focus is a one-to-one doctor/patient relationship, sanctified by confidentiality. Some medical professionals—particularly those in the mental health specialties—have begun to recognize that the patient is part of a complex family unit. I believe that as we accept the smallness of the world, the density of the population, and the myriad influences on individuals and families, someday we may recognize the community and even the whole society as the patient. Imagine, then, what a "doctor of society" might do, what kinds of diseases he or she might treat! Part of the Gesundheit Institute experiment is to be a doctor on all four levels—to the individual, the family, the community, and society—and see them as intensely interrelated.

The Key to a Happy Life

Do you see O my brothers and sisters? It is not chaos or death—it is form, union, plan—it is eternal life—it is Happiness."
Walt Whitman, "Song of Myself"

The most revolutionary act anyone can commit is to be happy. I refer not to a moment of joy during one of life's peak experiences but to a basic pattern of enduring happiness. It takes no greater effort to be happy every day than to be miserable.

Each of us chooses the background hues of his or her own portrait. A person can choose to be happy or miserable. Unfortunately, a paradigm of suffering and unhappiness seems to have dominated human awareness during the last five thousand years, with a basic, underlying feeling that life is a struggle. However, this could change and happiness could become the foundation from which life is launched. We can *choose* a paradigm of happiness in which all our thoughts, feelings, and actions are infused with joy.

Our culture's definition of happiness has made it an elusive goal, too closely associated with major events such as birthdays and weddings. Most of us are so habituated to pain that the concept of living happily *all the time* may seem impossible, even unnatural.

When we live our lives from a baseline of happiness, negative events still may happen. I am not speaking of a life without problems. On the contrary, sadness and unhappy feelings will occur in the larger context of a great and happy life. My hope is for each person to express such feelings freely, because unhappiness, once expressed, can recede into a paradigm of joy.

In my experience during the past thirty years, many people say they feel "sad all the time." Of course, they're not actually sad all the time, but it *feels* that way to them. The same applies to someone who is happy all the time: it *feels* that way. A defeatist attitude is a major part of the pain paradigm. Mozart was penniless, unable to find work, and sick. He had lost his children to starvation. Yet, while all of this happened, he wrote some of the most beautiful music ever created. It was not his genius that made him happy. For Mozart, happiness was an individual choice.

In our society the "gods" of money and power have made boredom, loneliness, and fear the context in which many of us live. Our news media—newspapers, TV, and radio—scream the headlines of pain each day. The news is slanted to cover the ugly, the tormented, the tragic. The camera dissects each traffic accident with surgical precision but reports happy news only in anecdotal asides. If I were to publish a newspaper, I would print mostly happy stories, relegating unhappy ones to the back pages, so that anyone who wanted to "make news" would have to do something funny. Imagine a newspaper that would ecstatically tell of a walk in the woods!

The focus on suffering permeates the popular culture as well. Splashy, commercial television productions promote negative emotions like suspicion, envy, and unhappiness. We have become so habituated to pain that many of us believe a happy existence would be undesirable or even boring. This is an interesting paradox. During years of in-depth conversations, I have learned that most people seek, even *pine* for, a happier life; yet many do not believe they can be continuously happy.

Part of the problem is the limited expression of happiness in the arts, especially in the twentieth century. In the visual arts, for example, advertising has become a repository of talent, largely because of its financial rewards. The few artists who work independently and speak from their hearts tend to paint a grim picture. I see very little current visual art that promotes the greatness of life. I am most familiar with the written arts, especially the novels, poetry, and drama of the last two centuries. The closest thing to a great, happy life in most literary works is the story of a hero who strives mightily to overcome adversity through love and diligence. This, however, is a struggle. Abysmally few authors sing of the joy of every single day. Walt Whitman does; in "Song of Myself" he wrote:

> *I celebrate myself, and sing myself,*
> *And what I assume you shall assume*
> *For every atom belonging to me as good belongs to you.*

Whitman expressed a universal vision in which life itself is great.

I am interested in happiness because I am a physician. Over the years, I have interviewed thousands of people extensively. Most say happiness is a rare commodity in their lives and can list the few specific times they were happy. People often decline to do things that would make them happy—a physician must completely ignore huge areas of a patient's life because the patient doesn't want to make lifestyle changes. With great sadness, we prescribe treatments that we know will only partly help.

Psychiatry is the science of the mind, but I have been unable to find even one paragraph devoted to happiness in a psychiatry text-book. I never hear medical professionals prescribing happiness to the mentally unhealthy, which, to me, means all who are unhappy. Journal ads promoting tranquilizers and "talk therapies" aim merely at helping patients *cope* with their problems. Only a paradigm of pain would accept such Lilliputian goals.

Many of us experience pain in relationships and the consequent effects on our mental and physical functioning. More than half of all marriages end in divorce. Stress from poor relationships can drive up blood pressure or exacerbate ulcers, back problems, drug abuse, and anxiety. As a doctor, I believe that *it does matter to your health to be happy.* It may be the most important health factor in your life. This link is well documented in Norman Cousins' *Head First.* To treat the illness and not the source of the pain—which is the relationship itself—is gross neglect. Confronting the pain is the domain of psychiatry and psychology. Psychiatrists can help explore every angle and possible cause of pain, but unless they also are "happiologists," they cannot help promote happiness—and better health.

Being happy has political implications. Peace and world cooperation belong to the happy paradigm, whereas wars and border disputes are part of the paradigm of pain. It is a trait of happiness to help others, just as it is a trait of pain to be lonely. Maybe if enough people become happy, the world could become more peaceful. Fun is what people have when they are happy. A single experience can provide fun. But when life is perceived as fun in all its aspects, the game of life becomes fun forever. This viewpoint does not trivialize the excitement of each moment; it simply makes wonder, curiosity, and enthusiasm pervasive. Let's look at some everyday occurrences that usually are seen as "downers," such as waiting in line. In the happy paradigm, waiting in line becomes a great opportunity to meet people, daydream, or play. Washing dishes—too often seen as drudgery— becomes a ballet performed in gratitude to the cook. Boredom is replaced by exploration. Our senses become our servants, ushering in a variety of interesting sights, sounds, and smells.

The most important ingredient in my personal recipe for happiness is my friends. Everybody needs friends or playmates with whom to have fun. In the pain paradigm, folks often say they're lucky to have a few friends. For the happy, however, every living soul offers that potential. The only lifetime relationship totally sanctioned by our society is marriage. Yet most who enter it rarely retain the element of play. All-too-serious jokes speak of marriage as loss of freedom. In the happy paradigm, marriage is the beginning of freedom. A limited perspective can keep love not only from lasting but from growing year by year.

Nothing in life can approach the breathtaking joy of the shared journey into parenthood. Could there possibly be a greater gift to a child than the parents' happiness with one another during the child's development? Today, the focus in marriage too often is on the struggle. The focus *could* be on the joy. Most relationships involve a large dose of both. Yet we hear far more about the pain because it seems to be associated with maturity. Enthusiastic joy is associated with childhood—as if it were something to outgrow.

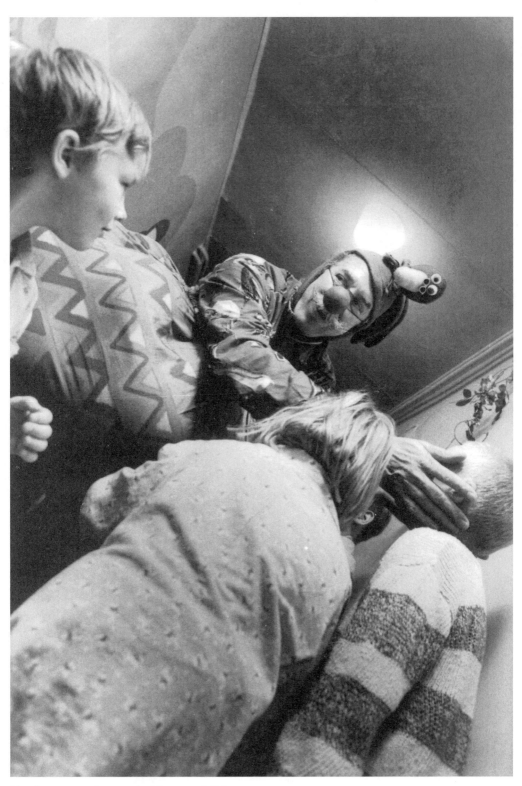

Patch at an orphanage in Moscow, 1996.

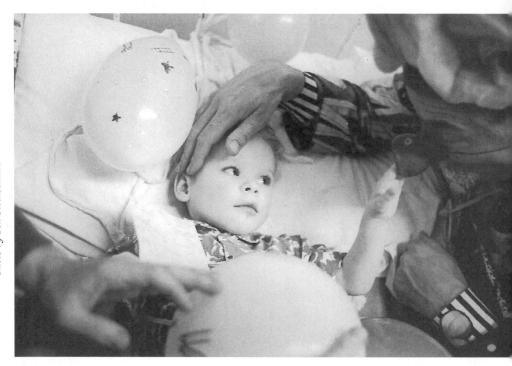

Patch at the bedside of a child with spinal tuberculosis at the Children's Hospital in St. Peter burg, 1996.

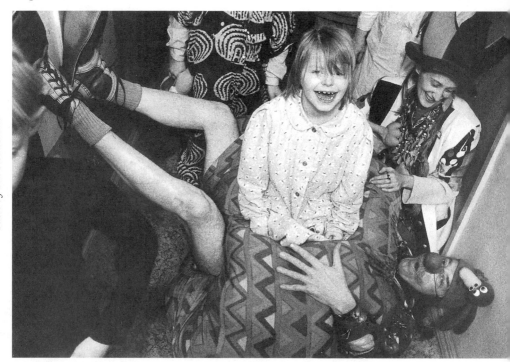

A Moscow orphan enjoys bouncing on Patch's balloon pants, 1996.

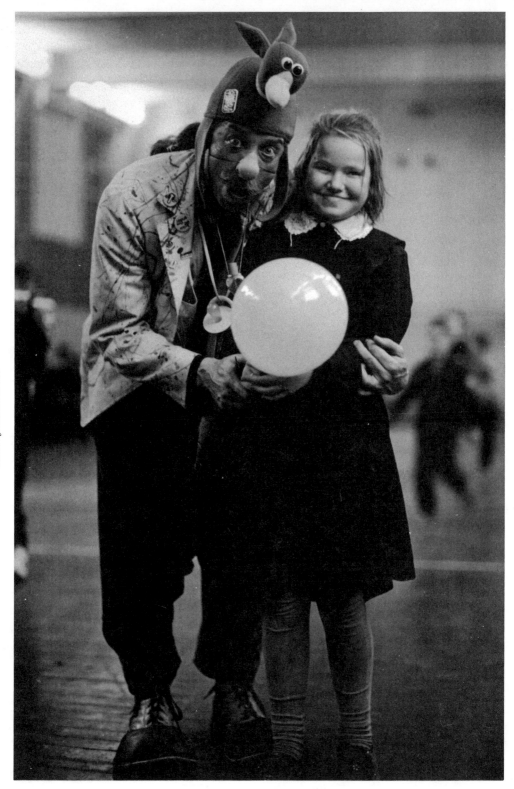

St. Petersburg Orphanage, 1991.

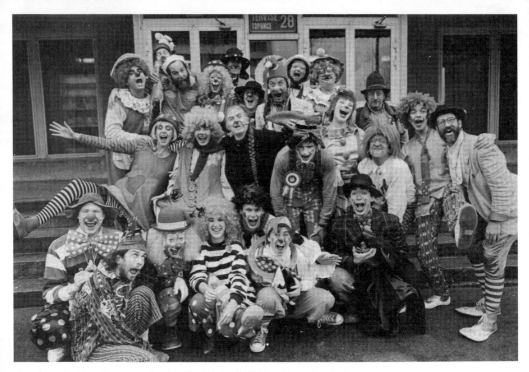

Patch and gang during a hospital visit in Tallinn, Estonia, 1991

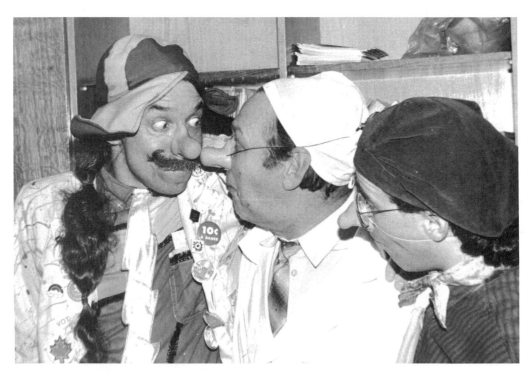

The head of the Children's Orthopedic Hospital in Pushkin, Russia, flanked by Patch and Mark Warren, another Gesundheit doctor, 1988.

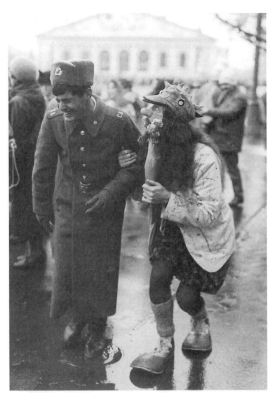
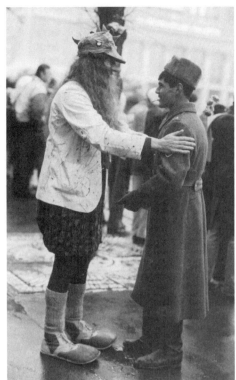
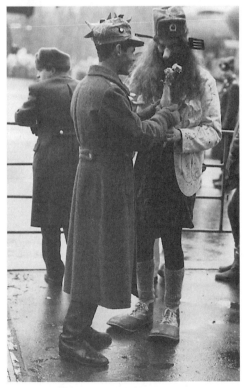
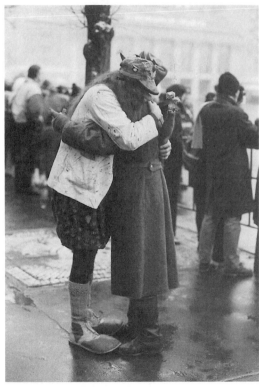

Patch with Russian soldiers at Moscow's Red Square, November 7, 1990—the last year of the military parade celebration of the 1917 Revolution.

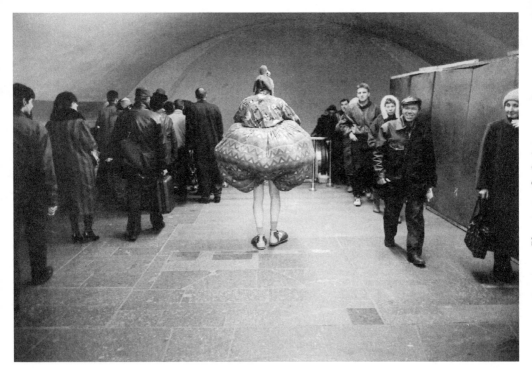

Patch goes for a walk in the Moscow Metro, 1996.

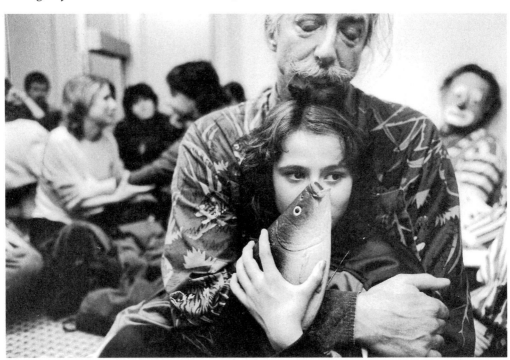

Patch holds Nadia, a Russian orphan, before saying good-bye, 1996.

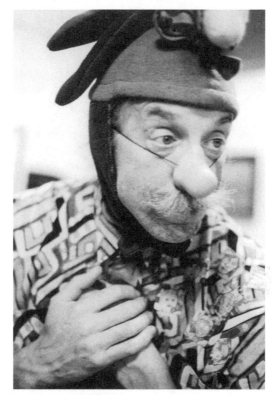

Photo by Ben Stechschulte

Patch at the Gesundheit Institute, 1996.

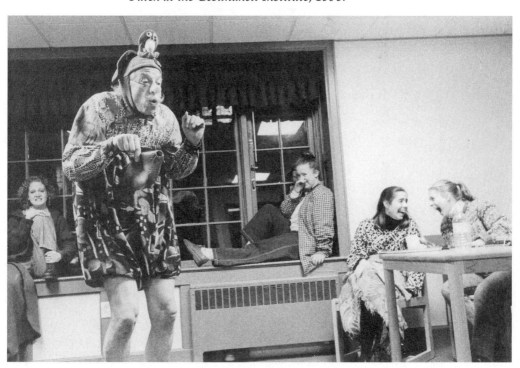

Patch clowning with freshmen students at Bucknell University, Lewisburg, Pennsylvania, 1996.

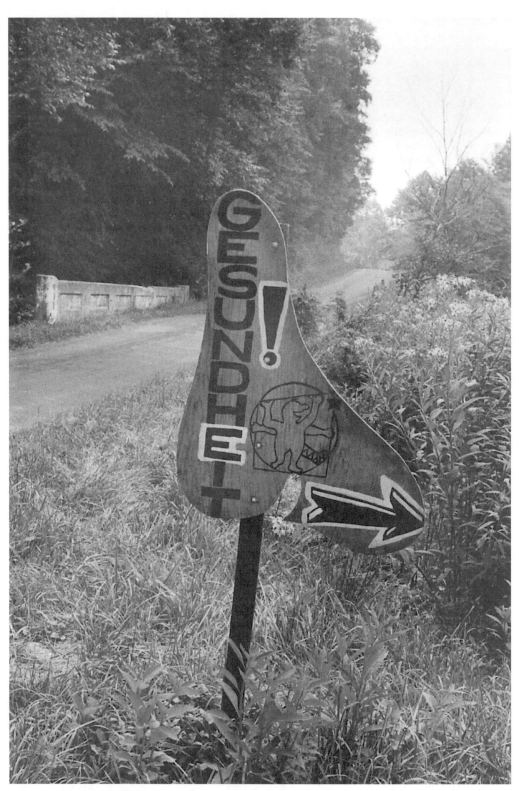

Road sign to the Gesundheit Institute in West Virginia.

What applies to lovers also is true of friends. The pain paradigm brings caution and suspicion to friendship. But if the seeds of trust are cultivated in a field of shared happiness, they will bloom forever. In a happier world, we would see a renaissance of extended families living together in mutual support. I have lived communally with happy groups for more than twenty years, and it has enriched my life and enhanced my dreams in every way. A large circle of friends can provide security and happiness in ways that no other form of insurance can.

Hobbies are also a key to a happy life; very simply, they are organized happiness, a personal decision to explore some particular aspect of life. Hobbies provide outlets for wonder and curiosity and even for our creative selves. In the paradigm of happiness, all of life's interests—including work and family—become hobbies. Robert Frost said in "Two Tramps in Mud-Time" that his goal in living was to make his vocation and avocation one.

People commonly abandon their interests when they feel sad or anxious. Yet this is the time to enlist the therapeutic value of hobbies. It is important to recognize the healing value of living our interests, whether we are sick or well. Usually, the choice of hobbies is immaterial as long as it doesn't hurt others. Most nonviolent hobbies are healing. Hobbies are our friends when we are alone and a vehicle for developing friendships when we are with others.

In the pain paradigm, nature becomes a servant to humanity's whims. This is a great tragedy. To the happy, however, nature is the sandbox of life. A rainy day is not dreary but a time for celebrating, for kinship with nature. Few things in life can approach the unabashed happiness that contemplating nature affords. To feel our feet on the grass or watch a hovering dragonfly or blooming plant is blissful. Nature is everywhere and it is free. For those who open their hearts to it, no day can pass without rapture.

Laughter is the white noise of happiness. A chuckle stands like a sentry at our consciousness, ready to burst out at the slightest provocation. Comic relief is a major way for happy folk to dissipate pain. In a healthier world, humor would be a way of life. People would be funny as a rule, not an exception. One of the best aids in the transition from a "heavy" to a "light" existence is to open up the comedian in oneself. People are hungry for humor, so if you can be silly around them, their thanks will garland your life.

It takes great effort to reject joy and beauty; it is not a passive act. With all the potential for happiness in this world, it is astounding that people are so bored and lonely. I do not intend to trivialize sadness or anxiety but simply to say that we choose these ways of life. People who feel sad tend to blame external events over which they have no control. This is irresponsible. Such individuals become accomplices to the paradigm of pain when they sing out the "script" of a victim. Yes, the terrible things that happen *are* painful. Choosing to give up, however, is what makes these experiences continue to wound us.

Viktor Frankl, a survivor of the Nazi concentration camps who knows the importance of freedom of choice, wrote:

> *We who lived in concentration camps can remember the men who walked through the huts comforting others, giving away their last piece of bread. They may have been few in number, but they offer sufficient proof that everything can be taken away from a man but one thing: the last of the human freedoms — to choose one's attitude in any given set of circumstances, to choose one's own way.*
>
> Viktor E. Frankl, *Man's Search for Meaning*

I am suggesting that even though the world's pain hurts us, we must keep love and peace in our lives. We must take every opportunity to shout "Whoopie!" Be an example of joy!

Friendship

In more than twenty years as a physician, I never have seen any suffering that begins to touch the horror of loneliness. The cries of this condition are gut-wrenching, and only friendship can really ease the pain. In conversations with people from all walks of life, I find that loneliness infects the vast majority. For many, loneliness is so paralyzing that it is a major deterrent to reaching out. Loneliness has become a private hell that the afflicted do not reveal unless probed deeply. Brief visits to the doctor or superficial conversations will not relieve their suffering. Acknowledging their emptiness is a vulnerability too painful to expose. For some people, loneliness manifests itself as immobility, for others as unbridled anger. But for everyone, loneliness is a horrible disease for which friendship is the best medicine.

For one human to love another: that is perhaps the most difficult of all of our tasks, the ultimate, the last test and proof, the work for which all other work is but preparation.
                                   Rainer Maria Rilke, *Letters to a Young Poet*

So often our parents and society make friendship seem *hard*. In our formative years we heard "You can count only on yourself" and "You can't trust other people." Youthful innocence opens up many friendships, but what happens in the ensuing years kills our innocence and capacity for friendship later in life. Shackled to the belief that "You're lucky to have one or two close friends," we rarely envision the possibility of hundreds. The deterioration of family, church, and tribal life has greatly aggravated this crisis of alienation. Yet, when I ask older people what matters in life, friendship ranks above all other factors put together.

What is a friend? A friend can be a playmate for life, certainly for the moment. Everything a person does goes better with friends. Do not confuse acquaintances with friends. Friendship is the blissful post-surrender relationship. A friend can be such a blessing that just the thought of him or her can bring smiles to one's face and peace to one's soul. Friends participate in each other's lives; one very special friend might become a bedmate and join with you to expand your circle of friends with children. A friend is a comfort, a confidant, an errand mate, a person to be yourself with. A friend soothes pain and fear. A friend tosses "yes" or "no" like juggling balls, giving them equal weight, in order to find truth, not to please. A friend says "yes," and your dreams come closer to reality.

It is unusual for a spouse or one friend to fulfill all one's chumship needs and share all one's physical, intellectual, and other interests. Nor should they be expected to. A variety of friendships reinforce one another and the primary spouse/friend relationship.

How can you become a friend or be ready to receive friendship? The desire for friendship must be intense. If your friends come first, your actions must show it. Touch with your eyes and body on every possible occasion. Think of your friends every day, and tell them of your love and appreciation. Respect to your core the fact that you need them. Never doubt your friendships and never hold back on them. Never play the debit-and-credit game. The value of a gift can never surpass that ultimate gift of friendship—freedom from loneliness. To preserve your friendships:

- Surround yourself with pictures and mementos of your friends at home and at work. They are icons for the soul.

- Listen to your friends' dreams and make them yours in every way possible.

- Always feel that you're doing your best. Guilt has no place in friendship.

- If a potential friend has an interest, say, "Yes, I'll try." Few things initiate friendship as quickly as adopting another's interest.

- Penetrate into their lives and reveal your deepest feelings freely. Express a desire for comfort.

- Preserve your friendships with a postcard, letter, or phone call. Long-distance friendships are easy to maintain. Be aggressive.

- Give friends shelter and support. Move from the insurance of cash to the insurance of clan.

- Play with each other every time you're together.

- Need your friends not in desperation but in anticipation.

Friends are not hard to make. There is an unlimited supply of people of every imaginable sort. Shop around uninhibitedly. Those who radiate joy, gentleness of spirit, and a humility of need will cultivate only a fraction of the great friendships that come their way.

> To be the recipient of affection is a potent cause of happiness, but the man who demands affection is not the man upon whom it is bestowed. The man who receives affection is, speaking broadly, the man who gives it.
>
> Bertrand Russell, *The Conquest of Happiness*

Friendship bestows more than happiness—it is the best medicine ever discovered! Treasure friendship, celebrate it, make it the central focus of life, and enjoy the most secure form of health insurance.

I Give: Surrendering Can Set You Free

When I was a kid we did a lot of male wrestling and fighting—some playful, some painful. In either case, when I felt overpowered, I would say, "I give." It was a chance to display my meekness. In "giving," I surrendered my will to the power that won. I relaxed my muscles and felt a lot calmer. It made great sense never to fight again—or at least to try. I wondered how to lessen the number of fights involving both me and other people. I surrendered to the strength and skill of the winner, knowing that I could sustain that calm by never thinking I could win a fight and by "giving" before it ever started. I enjoyed the surrender. It made me feel true to myself.

In adulthood, I learned that all those seemingly "outside" fights actually were going on inside my head, but they were a lot more complex. There were too many combatants, in fact, to count even a fraction of them. I'm sure these inner combats caused the two duodenal ulcers I had at the age of seventeen and ultimately led to the suicide attempts and hospitalization. For many years, I could not respond "I give" to these inner battles. In the mental hospital, my friends came to visit me. At the end of my tether, I finally realized that only in surrendering to the depths of friendship could I find the calm I was seeking. I needed friends! At last, I discovered my soul in their hands. It felt great.

> No man is an Iland, intire of it selfe; every man is a peece of the
> Continent, a part of the maine, if a Clod bee washed away by the
> Sea, Europe is the lesse, as well as if a Promontorie were, as well as
> if a Mannor of thy friends or If thine owne were; any mans death
> diminishes me, because I am involved in Mankinde; And therefore
> never send to know for whom the bell tolls; It tolls for thee.
>
> John Donne, *Devotions*

The process of surrender seemed easier after I learned what is essential to my life and gave it full attention. By essential, I mean anything that is completely free of doubt. Surrender is not an on/off phenomenon but a dynamic relationship with an infinite number of factors. One can have a dramatic impact on many of these factors and take an active part in calming oneself.

Most adults I meet harbor a huge amount of doubt and an inability to surrender. A remarkably large number of people perceive that they have nothing to surrender to, no sheltering umbrella of belief. Life rarely is a vibrant joy. Paradoxically, they have surrendered, instead, to despair, loneliness, and fear. This kind of negative surrender is disturbingly prevalent and profound.

"The Woman at the Washington Zoo"

The saris go by me from the embassies.

Cloth from the moon. Cloth from another planet.
They look back at the leopard like the leopard.
And I . . .
this print of mine, that has kept its color
Alive through so many cleanings; this dull null
Navy I wear to work, and wear from work, and so
To my bed, so to my grave, with no
Complaints, no comment: Neither from my chief,
The Deputy Chief Assistant, nor his chief—
Only I complain. . . . this serviceable
Body that no sunlight dyes, no hand suffuses
But, dome-shadowed, withering among columns,
Wavy beneath fountains—small, far-off shining
In the eyes of animals, these beings trapped
As I am trapped, but not themselves, the trap,
Aging, but without knowledge of their age,
Kept safe here, knowing not of death, for death—
Oh, bars of my own body, open, open!

The world goes by my cage and never sees me.
And there come not to me as come to these,
The wild beasts, sparrows pecking the llamas' grain,
Pigeons settling on the bears' bread, buzzards
Tearing the meat the flies have clouded. . . .

Vulture,
When you come for the white rat that the foxes left,
Take off the red helmet of your head, the black
Wings that have shadowed me, and step to me as man:

The wild brother at whose feet the white wolves fawn,
To whose hand of power the great lioness
Stalks purring. . . .

You know what I was,
you see what I am: change me, change me!

Randall Jarrell

Regrettably, surrender can serve despair and evil just as passionately as it serves good. History constantly reminds us of those who surrender to war as a pleasure. The 1991 war in the Persian Gulf is a sad case in point. How does anybody surrender to killing? Where is the creativity to solve complex problems? This war made me shed tears. People seemed cautious before the war: it was unpopular. But after the first exciting night of bombing, reported with all the lingo of the Superbowl, January 17, 1991, became a day of rejoicing. A glorious superiority, felt as nationalism, blossomed along with widespread surrender to the idea of war. The only time TV ever drops regular programming that long is for the great TV glue: horror. What kind of positive event—what glorious cornucopia of fun and love—must occur to stop regular TV programming for 48 hours?

Over time, surrender has become part of my life: surrender to simple hobbies, music, pets, or the delicious pastimes of fun and play. The more I surrender to fun and play, the more they become as important as love in creating my personal calm. Paradoxically, the more I surrender the stronger I feel. Surrender has ceased to be helplessness and has become survival wisdom.

I believe that faith is the most important single factor in one's well-being. In this context the nature of faith is immaterial; the key is the degree of surrender and commitment to belief. Once that depth is reached—free of doubt and full of celebration—the potential for joy is immense. To approach a person with such faith is to bathe in the ocean. Surrender empowers action in whatever direction belief takes it. The phrase *I give* implies surrender—and the action that comes with surrender: service.

Community: Medicine for Life

For more than a million years, human primates have lived in tribes. I'm sure we came together for mutual interdependence in child rearing, security, and food gathering. The fun of being part of a collective came as a powerful secondary benefit. This drive to huddle together, I am convinced, became part of our genetic coding. When we changed from a hunting-gathering to an agricultural society, the traveling band divided to claim individual plots of land and began to huddle in households and villages. As villages grew into cities, huddling happened in neighborhoods. As we moved farther apart, communities diminished to become extended families, then nuclear families, and finally solitary dwellings. The arts, psychology, and sociology characterize this progression as the alienation of society.

During many years of doctoring, I have found few people with a circle of deeply committed friends. Indeed, the vast majority of individuals feel lucky to have a few "close acquaintances." Ultimately, life goes better with a circle of friends. Without this circle of safety, it is extremely difficult to erase the fear that pervades the economy, health care system, relationships, and other aspects of life. This fear must be cast aside to foster the surrendering required to form a community.

Community can be experienced in many forms. I speak not of membership cards or notations on a resume, but of commitment to individuals through action. The form of community that I love dearly, in which I have lived for more than twenty years, has been the most significant factor in furthering all my dreams, both personal and professional.

Living in community can help keep relationships vibrant and strong. If you're surrounded by friends, you have many options when you want a playmate, some deep conversation, or help with the chores. If your partner is tied up with a project, you can just invite a housemate to be with you. Every communal meal can be a dinner party with conversation sizzling. When you share work, each person may cook one night a week, infrequently enough to put heart and soul into the meal. Shared cleaning duties too are sporadic enough to be enjoyable. And child rearing is the best of all. In community, children have magical input from many people who share not only their time but their talents, personalities, and wisdom.

Professionally, communal life has allowed me to chase many rainbows. Gesundheit Institute could not have progressed as far as it has if it were the quest of one man. But with group living, Gesundheit is the by-product of many friends' commitment. I cannot conceive of practicing medicine in today's context, and only the grace of community allows me to live as I do. By sharing costs and possessions, we have been able to do big things for pennies. For eight years, all of the costs of operating the building site in West Virginia have been paid by donations. We are slowly building a community of supporters throughout the United States who are sending what they can to build our hospital.

My personal growth also has been enhanced by community. I grad-uated from medical school "head smart." While living in community, however, I have built buildings, farmed, raised goats, produced movies, and learned rope walking and unicycling. Even these achievements are dwarfed by the happiness I feel amid so many friends. This security transcends economics.

How can one begin to take steps toward community? First, be ready to belong with all your heart and soul. Examine current relationships and dare to dream of what their potential might be. The better defined the dreams, the happier the journey. Those who see the dream as a journey, and not as a final product, can realize it in the present and not in the future.

Community will not sustain itself casually. It requires patience and flexibility, virtues that remove many hurdles. For example, if a group makes rules everybody didn't vote for, the dissenters should give their active support without grumbling. Patience and flexibility, backed by similar goals, can make a marriage or a community work. Consider making this level of commitment. It is scary, but deep commitment will make community and friendships attainable.

This marriage of friends in community will be the most complex and difficult thing most people will ever do. Study the field; much practical information on relationships and community is available. Also, try to analyze relationships to learn what works and what doesn't. How do dishes get done? How does the hammer get back to its proper place? The greater the commitment, the easier the task. Be a self-starter and let the joy of labor be its own reward. Do the work of two or three people, not competitively but in the excitement of serving the extended family. Find ways to love the jobs others hate—be a family trouble-shooter. Be sure to play with each community member; the broader one's contacts within the group, the warmer its blanket of security. When every group member becomes a playmate, each issue becomes everybody's issue. Many communities get into trouble because they don't value group play as much as they value group work.

Other important factors must be considered in creating a happy community life, and each group must juggle them to come up with their own approach. Many people who are interested have written to me. I promise to act as a resource person and to share ideas or information on references beyond those listed in the bibliography.

We Are All One Family

A plague in our society has struck all income levels and social classes and threatens our future security. No medication can eradicate it, and no vaccine or immunization can prevent it. This plague, the breakdown of the family, is symptomatic of an unhealthy society; it can be arrested only by aggressive efforts to change societal trends.

Bringing up children presents one of life's greatest challenges. Even in the happiest of marriages it is the most time-consuming, gut-wrenching task a person can undertake. It is not surprising that tribes and extended families have made child raising a group effort. In the United States the nuclear family has failed at this responsibility. More than half of all marriages now end in divorce, and many that survive are not mutually fulfilling. This situation has created legions of single-parent households.

It is inconceivable that so many people try to raise children by themselves. Single parents are truly the greatest heroes of our modern era. I salute their valiant efforts. These jugglers attempt to be mother, father, wage earner, social organizer, and hobby chairperson all at once. Many end up needing medical care as a result of the stresses of this arduous task.

One way to support their efforts is to help them recreate an extended "family." Many single parents—and others—could escape their loneliness with compatible roommates. If we try to know all our patients intimately, we will find many who have extra rooms in their homes. By having a parent and children live with them, these generous people could find their lives enriched by the companionship, by the environmental stimulation, and above all by the joy of service to humanity. Band together!

In the long term, to solve the problem of single parenting, we should encourage our educational system to teach students about relationships and communication. If family life is one of our most important life journeys, it seems wise to teach young people how to increase the chances of having a happy family. As holistic doctors, we must value loving human relationships and interdependent community living, which are essential to the health of the whole person and are factors that we can change.

I am not implying that something is wrong with the single parent. Many women, unhappy in their relationships with men, choose to have children without a father; other women's pregnancies are less voluntary. People should not necessarily stay in unhealthy relationships unless they are trying to improve them. I'm suggesting that both parent and child need support, whether the source is single or paired, male, female, or community based. I'm suggesting that individuals and groups who want to give service can make no greater contribution than to help the single parent.

Choosing Wellness

Exercise and recreation . . . are as necessary as reading: I will rather say more necessary, because health is worth more than learning.
Thomas Jefferson, letter to John Garland Jefferson, 1790

Building a happy, connected life can have wonderful empowering benefits. Just as we can choose to be happy or to reach out to others, we can choose to be healthy. In medical school, health was defined as the absence of disease, so people not complaining of symptoms were "healthy." Few adults I've spoken with, though, describe life as a wondrous, zestful journey. Most illnesses a family doctor sees have a huge lifestyle component. This frustrates the physician because the illnesses could have been prevented with self-care.

Obviously, health is far more than a disease-free interlude. To be healthy is to have a body toned to maximum performance potential, a clear mind exploding with wonder and curiosity, and a spirit at peace with the world. Most adults, however, exist in a gray area between health and sickness, a zone in which they say "I'm fine" when asked how they feel. This "fine" can be a cover for all kinds of dis-ease: the fatigue and "blah" feeling experienced by those sensitive to fluctuations in blood sugar as a result of a high-sugar diet; the foot problems that come from wearing shoes geared for fashion, not fitness; the distraction and anger that linger after poor communication with a spouse or friend. In fact, there are hundreds of silent ways our lifestyle assaults us and anticipates future expression in disease.

In the future I predict that simply enduring life and feeling "fine" will no longer be satisfactory for the healthy. Like Walt Whitman, we will "sing the body electric." A movement is afoot within the healing arts and education to fill the great void of health care. Members of this movement say that life is extremely complex and the way we experience it is intimately tied to our lifestyles. In other words, how we live determines how healthy we are. Many lifestyle factors are so powerful that by attending to just a few, we can feel surges of health. The term *wellness* encompasses everything that affects how we feel, the interconnectedness of these factors, and all efforts to translate them into action.

Wellness is the sum of everything that makes us healthier. In the wellness model, patients become responsible for their own health. The health care professional's role shifts from that of mechanic fixing a breakdown to a gardener nurturing growth, because wellness results from active participation that only the self can give.

Wellness is an investment with many payoffs. A long-term commitment to good health leads to a lifetime of high-quality living for the investor. A body in tone and at proper weight allows a person to indulge every wish for activity, not limiting it because he or she is out of shape. But the benefits of wellness extend far beyond the self, affecting family and work as well. Family life can become creative and rich in communication and cooperation. People who are in maximum health can be happier and more loving in all their relationships. The workplace also can become more enjoyable if caring and curiosity help make every employee a team member and every task a delight. An individual striving to be healthy brings loving management and creativity to the workplace. Studies have shown that emphasizing a human-centered, healthy workplace and providing space and time to exercise cuts absenteeism and turnover and increases productivity. So it's even profitable to be healthy!

Unfortunately, one of life's ironies is that wisdom comes mostly with age. By the time we realize that a habit has profoundly harmed us, we feel helpless to change it. We may even justify it as intrinsic to our nature. Luckily, the design of the human organism is such that it can recover remarkably well; in fact, it begins to repair itself as soon as we alter an unhealthy habit.

Life is a cascade of choices, and we are an expression of both the short-term and long-term choices we make. To cut back on the number of decisions made daily, we fall into habits in which a routine substitutes for a choice. Still, a habit can be a double-edged sword, because once entrenched it is incredibly hard to break, especially when it is an unhealthy one. Wellness, in a sense, is a system to help people restructure habits to make their lifestyles healthier, not by making great effort but simply by adopting positive, intentional habits.

Take *nutrition*, for example. To simplify human physiology, we are a sack of water containing chemicals in solution. How those chemicals interact determines what we are. But in many interactions, chemicals are used up or altered and must be replenished. Nutrition consists of the proper consumption and assimilation of foods containing chemicals the body needs. Since few foods contain all or most of these nutrients, we must obtain them from a variety of foods.

As people have moved farther from food sources, and food companies have processed their products to have a longer shelf life, our diets have changed dramatically. For the last 100 years or more, synthetic chemicals, refined foods, sugar, and salt have replaced many of the natural foods our ancestors ate. Laboratory rats that would have thrived on the heavy dark breads of our ancestors now die when fed commercial bread. Refined simple sugars are ubiquitous in our daily lives. At the turn of the century, we consumed three pounds of sugar per person per year; now we consume more than 125 pounds per person annually. Many scientists propose that sugar consumption has had a profound effect on our health; certainly, it plays a major role in one of the most devastating of diseases: obesity. The federal government has stepped in to encourage new nutritional habits, including dramatic cutbacks in sugar and salt intake, increases in foods containing fiber, and vast decreases in milk and other animal fat products. I would add these guidelines: eat mostly whole grains, fresh fruits and vegetables, and, for non-vegetarians, fish and poultry rather than red meat. Other approaches to good nutrition include learning to cook healthy foods, growing one's own vegetables to experience the labor and joy of fresh produce, and reading labels on packaged foods to avoid those containing chemicals that can be disruptive to our genes.

If nutrition is the fuel, *exercise* is the toner for the body. Modern civilization has changed few things as drastically as the amount of exercise we get. We have never been as sedentary as we are today. This, combined with high-calorie sugar and fat intake, has made large segments of our adult population overweight and flabby. A law in biology says "Use it or lose it." The interplay of muscles, bones, tendons, ligaments, and joints demands consistent stimulation to stay in tone. Being in shape does not mean simply being slender but having all the muscles trained.

There are four kinds of exercise to consider. The body's internal toner is *heart-lung (aerobic) exercise* that strengthens the heart, exercises the lungs (to supply oxygen and rid the body of carbon dioxide), and tones muscles used in physical activity. All of these give the body endurance. *Stretching* or *yoga-style exercises* keep the body's joints and muscles limber and relaxed. *Strength exercises* are important to tone muscles not affected by heart-lung exercises. *Balancing exercises* like dance, gymnastics, or circus skills add yet another dimension to maximum performance. Being in shape has hidden benefits as well. Exercise can lower blood pressure, enhance mental health, diminish adverse reactions to stress, and aid digestion. I believe regular exercise may slow the aging process as well.

Just as we exercise our bodies to be fit, so must we exercise our minds to keep alert. The greatest instruments for mental stimulation are *wonder* and *curiosity*. Boredom is a major disease, eroding the health of many adults who, over time, narrow their spheres of interest. Wonder and curiosity are tools all young children possess. In fact, they are what make kids seem so alive. For many adults, sunsets have become routine and life's pace too hectic. But wonder and curiosity can be recaptured! No stimulant can awaken a person like a new and captivating interest or an ongoing exploration. The next time a friend or family member is excited about something, jump in and share that interest. Carry wonder and curiosity into old age, and they will preserve your youthfulness. Often, a vibrant interest is a major motivation for staying healthy because good health allows the exploration to continue.

Love is the most important way to sustain a healthy, happy life.

This passionate abstraction has captivated artists, who have attempted to define and elucidate it. We most commonly express love toward family, friends, God, self, lovers, pets, nature, or hobbies. Love is unconditional surrender to the overwhelming feeling experienced when giving or receiving it. By surrender, I mean loss of oneself in awe, trust, respect, enjoyment, and tenderness toward the object of surrender. The more one submits to unconditional love toward one object, the easier it becomes to submit to unconditional love for others. The unconditional aspect is vitally important: without it, love is often killed by expectations, doubts, and fears.

The study of love is no longer the exclusive realm of the artist. Scientists now have conclusive evidence that it is the most important stress-reducing force known, just as loss or lack of love is the most potent disease-promoting force. These studies are explained in *Love, Medicine & Miracles* by Dr. Bernie Siegel, a surgeon at Yale. If love is the foundation for happiness, then fun, play, and laughter are the vehicles for its expression. The great physician Sir William Osler said that laughter is the "music of life." And one of humor's important psychological functions is to transform old habits into new perspectives and behaviors.

Faith is the cornerstone of our inner strength, a personal, passionate belief in something of inexhaustible power and mystery. Whenever we must face any devastating change without some kind of solid belief, we become prey to confusion, fear, and panic. Often these crises raise questions that have no answers. The pain arising from this uncertainty is healed by our beliefs. Faith has no physical characteristics, no external requirements. It's not a commodity. In order to acquire a belief, one simply needs to have the interest and willingness to submit to its mystery. Although many fine religions promote a common interpretation of belief, I think that each person must find an individual, meaningful faith. Faith is not a label but an inner experience of strength that lives in each person, day by day. Dr. Scott Peck has explored in depth the relationship between faith and health in his popular book *The Road Less Traveled*.

While faith is intangible, *nature* is a physical, sensual thing. Our relationship with nature throughout history has been part of a healthy life. It is not surprising that most symbols in early religions came from nature. Our moods often are described in terms of nature. A synonym for "happy" is "sunny." The first warm, bright day after winter raises spirits as few other days can. Likewise, love has a metaphorical connection to the moon. Most of our early celebrations grew out of the seasons. We have such strong needs to connect with nature that we spend billions of dollars to bring it home in the form of pets and houseplants. Medical literature currently is saturated with accounts of the therapeutic benefits of pets for the elderly and mentally ill. Flowers are a universal way to communicate love at sickbeds, deaths, marriages, birthdays, and other special events. Our few weeks of vacation each year are mostly spent at the beach, in the mountains, or in other natural settings. Nature, after all, is the mother of wonder. If we are to be healthy, we need daily communion with both the spectacular sunset and the hardy blade of grass that pushes up through the sidewalk.

Another major wellness factor is *creativity*. Life is experienced as a rich journey if our imaginations, hands, and senses are tools for creating. Creativity is expressed not just through hobbies and art, but through our work, our families, and even how we wait in line. The process is more important than the final product. Creativity works like muscles: the more it is exercised, the greater its tone. Just as sitting in front of a television set all day atrophies mental and physical muscles, consistent passive entertainment kills creativity. Passivity can be countered by exploring new ideas and activities, never settling for one point of view. The key here is to be open and spontaneous. Don't catalog hobbies and interests as indulgences; rather, respect them as major medicines.

As soon as people recognize how fortunate they are to be well, the urge to give thanks arises. The healthy way to express gratitude is through *service*. Unless individuals have given some form of service, I believe that it will be difficult for them to feel that life is ultimately fulfilling. John Donne wrote "No man is an Iland" to acknowledge that we all are connected in some way. Only by helping others can we discover deep interdependence. It is vital that service be performed out of thanks and the joy of giving, because service easily can give rise to a debit/credit mentality. Service can take many forms: being a loving friend, helping a stranger in need, strengthening the community one lives in.

The world has grown smaller, so that our actions affect others even at great distances. It is impossible to separate individual wellness from that of our society or planet. To be truly healthy, we must use our creative talents to attain social and global change. It is imperative that we regard world peace as attainable and work to achieve it. We must cast off fear and doubt and learn to love and care for all people without waiting for others to take the first step. We must take an active role in local, state, and national politics, insisting on candidates who will help create a healthy society and world. The point is to act.

I have briefly touched on some major aspects of healthy living. There are many more. Wellness is not a fad. It is life insurance in the truest sense of the word. To live a healthy life means living at maximum potential in order to benefit oneself and one's work, family, and society. Health is the greatest of all assets, but it cannot be purchased or hoarded. Wellness is a process, a journey during which we choose which paths to follow. We cannot depend on health gained in the past; it must be renewed each day.

Huge · What Happens to a Dream Unleashed?

Huge means spending every day in zestful expression of one's highest self.

First, I'd like to introduce some of my friends: immense, vast, enormous, astronomical, tremendous, prodigious, stupendous, larger-than-life, infinite, mammoth, mastodonic, gigantic, gargantuan, Herculean, Atlantean, jumbo, humongous, whopping, whacking, thumping, thundering, and BIG!

I'm talking about a word so vivacious that grammarians give it its own punctuation—the exclamation point. Try to tame it—HUGE! One can't imagine "more huge." In the inanimate world, "huge" is simply the biggest. In the animate world, it is expressed as passion. For me, huge means intoxicating vision, daring to look at the miracle of life and dream without inhibition. It means to look at yourself and decide that death is the only limiting factor, and that maybe even death can be used to good purpose. Huge means spending every day in zestful expression of one's highest self. Skepticism be damned! Failures become the building blocks for the next step. End results may loom large, but true largeness resides in the exuberant effort spent getting there.

> *This is my quest, to follow that star*
> *no matter how hopeless, no matter how far*
> *to fight for the right, without question or pause*
> *to be willing to march into hell for a heavenly cause.*
> Dale Wasserman, *Man of La Mancha*

Huge can be applied to every part of one's life. The most personal is friendship: dreaming of and creating the most enriching relationships with the people one meets. Fundamental to achieving friendship is feeling the huge in oneself and loving one's very being. I'm not sure huge can happen if this feeling doesn't develop. This huge of other people makes me love cities so much, for here is where most people live. Crowded streets and lines of people become strings of pearls. I can imagine how unique each person is and how knowing them would embellish my life. Huge is trying to feel the friendship of every co-traveler on the planet.

> *You've got to have a dream, if you don't have a dream,*
> *how you gonna have a dream come true?*
> Oscar Hammerstein II, *South Pacific*

I revel in the hugeness of personal interests and hobbies. Life offers infinite choices. They exist in people's gardens and in their bowling games. What about Darwin's voluminous writings on barnacles? *The Guinness Book of World Records,* a tip of the iceberg, delights multitudes of voyeurs surveying other people's huge-ability. I love these individual expressions of human variation; they stimulate my own. One of my goals is to juggle fire while riding a unicycle in my gorilla costume on a slack rope. I have almost all the pieces ready and need only to combine them. Some dreams, perhaps many, will never be completed. For example, I would love to meet and play with everybody in the world. I would love to read all the books ever written. But who cares if I don't? It's the effort that satisfies me.

When your heart is in your dreams,
no request is too extreme . . .
when you wish upon a star,
your dreams come true.
  Ned Washington and Leigh Harline, *Pinocchio*

An important huge is the way a person expresses thanks for being alive. The person who does so through service will possess a great comfort throughout life. Huge encompasses world peace, an end to hunger, and harmony with nature. We must tackle these dreams in concert with all the world's workers; only a huge collective can make them happen. Within that framework, anything is possible. Jean Giano wrote *The Man Who Planted Trees* about a quiet, gentle man who during his lifetime single-handedly replanted many square miles of trees, at his own expense, on land he did not own. I think that this kind of effort represents the fountain of youth sought by so many. Service is one of the greatest medicines ever discovered. It is the great fatigue killer, the destroyer of depression and boredom, the way to end immobility caused by fear. As H. D. Thoreau said in *Walden*, "If you have built castles in the air, your work need not be lost; that is where they should be."

Huge is not for the whiner or the impatient. Huge does not belong to the casual person who goes with the flow. Huge *is* the flow. Huge has great respect for *being here now*, yet knows that large events are composed of small details. One does not win or inherit huge. Anybody can have it. Huge is a fabulous addiction or a heavenly codependence. Huge is romance in its fullest sense.

I extend appreciation to all who follow their dreams, whatever they may be, whether in the healing arts or other endeavors. Every patient I have met who has transcended suffering—despite severe chronic disease, intractible pain, or impending death—has had "huges." Most of them have had many.

PART II

A Prescription
for Health
and Healing

Health care in the United States is sick and in danger of dying. All of us know it. Prominent medical journals devote articles and editorials to fixing the system or finding alternatives; politicians base their campaign platforms on health care issues. The poor suffer most of all. But the discussions of "solutions" don't get to the root of the problem: the existing system focuses on sickness, not wellness, and health care costs too much and is available to too few.

What is needed is a drastic rethinking of the problem. Rather than trying to quick-fix the crumbling health care system, we need to create solutions that will excite both patients and caregivers. We must, in a mutual, multidisciplinary effort, tear down what hurts us and go on to heal a profession of healers. We must take medicine out of the business sector and recognize that greed and selfishness have placed society—and its health care system—in great peril. Our citizens need to feel a sense of belonging and of community. By attending to all members of society, improved health care could help unite society.

Gesundheit Institute is one group's vision of how this can be done. We've come a long way since the original thought, back in the early 1970s, that we wanted to love patients. Now, with our plans in the works for a new, fun, home-style hospital, we're focusing in a more serious way. We are committed to building a community that embodies to the extreme the philosophy that art, fun, and connectedness are as important to health as CAT scans and IVs. We want to act as a stimulus to others to create their own ideal medical community and to provide an example that others can follow, at least to some small degree.

Throughout our evolution, we have never separated the individual, community, and global levels. The ultimate goal of Gesundheit Institute is to address the greatest health issue of our time: world peace. We believe that the changes people make toward greater health are also steps toward world harmony. Our collective progress so far with quitting smoking and wearing seat belts is just a warm-up for disarmament. What if there were sustained peace on earth? What are the side effects of an abundance of fun? Our ambitions are limitless as we explore new ways to embrace health.

This section of the book traces the evolution of the Gesundheit dream, from the early days when, for want of a better name, people called us "the Zanies" ("Gesundheit Institute" wasn't coined until 1979), to the present, as we work to build our model facility in West Virginia. As a reflection of the communal nature of this project, the voices of a few of the people who have brought Gesundheit Institute to its present state also are heard here.

A Chronology of the Gesundheit Institute

1971: Our first house at 1318 N. George Mason Drive. Internship—the beginnings of loving patients, using humor and fun therapeutically. I decide to become a general practitioner.

1972–1973: 1202 N. Danville Street, Arlington, Virginia. First garden; deep exploration into performing arts; first full-time facility. I stay at home in a stunning hive of activity. First real time to be a *family* doctor. Realize prevention forefront. First encounter with alternative therapies. Acupuncturist practices in basement.

1973–1974: Europe trip—a book in itself. Fifteen people live in each other's company for eleven months on a large bus in Europe, Africa, and Russia. Intended to make relationships so tight that they could withstand all pressures of the next step.

1974–1977: 3661 West Ox Road, our most distinct pilot project. The same fifteen people (minus a few) plus up to twenty folk live on twelve acres. We doctors see 500 to 1,000 people at house per month. We live in a six-bedroom house, with two-acre farm, outdoor stage—a wild extravaganza. My first child is delivered at home.

1977–1979: The Rocks, West Virginia. We buy eighty-acre farm. Last active year. See people from forty states and eighteen foreign countries. Idyllic setting, but support staff slowly shows burnout from lack of privacy, no facility. I eventually must decide to leave (or fight, which is not in me). We have been together from 1971 to 1979 but realize that to continue, we must have a facility.

1979–1981: Herndon, Virginia. While James "J. J." Johnson, the doctor who's been with me from beginning, helps defuse The Rocks, I move nearer to D.C. to devote more time to fund-raising. I reorganize. Many doctors and nurses are ready to join up. I have time for more outreach. Linda and I goat farm with twenty goats. Buy 310-acre farm in Pocahontas County, West Virginia.

1981–present: Arlington, Virginia. Decide to take further step closer to D.C. Gareth Branwyn and Pam Bricker move in to devote time to fund-raising and to publish a newsletter. Gradually stop seeing patients as I choose to accept publicity, begin doing lectures, workshops. Receive in excess of $1 million from wealthy individuals and foundations, but mostly from plain folks. Begin building facility in West Virginia as some people live on the land.

6 • The Pilot Period

People often ask, "How did you earn a living if you weren't charging your patients?"

What we call the pilot period roughly spans the years from 1971 to 1983. Throughout this time, we experimented not only with ways of practicing medicine but also with living in community and learning to enjoy life and one another. After my short-lived residency, I set up a medical practice at home, a house I shared with three or four friends in Arlington, Virginia. Having guests overnight seemed to bond people, so we always encouraged people to stay and had a full house. Dancing together seemed to bond people, so we did that, too. It was our first communal experiment. The next year, six to eight of us moved to 1202 North Danville Street in Arlington. The bedrooms were tiny, but we had room for a garden and lots of visitors. Here we started our first full-time medical facility and began not charging our patients or accepting third-party reimbursement, refusing to carry malpractice insurance, and emphasizing preventive medicine and alternative therapies. As it turned out, we continued these practices.

During this period I met another doctor, James "J. J." Johnson, who remains my partner and a vital part of Gesundheit Institute. He had recently completed a year of residency in internal medicine and family practice and had quit in disgust. He then did alternative service at St. Elizabeth's Public Health Service Hospital in Washington instead of going into the military. One day, a classmate of mine from medical school, who also was doing alternative service at St. Elizabeth's, brought J. J. over, thinking we would like him. I loved him right away. We began working together and he has been an integral part of Gesundheit Institute ever since.

Two years out of medical school, I already had seen hundreds of patients, mostly young people interested in alternative lifestyles. Who else would go to a long-haired doctor in 1971? The counterculture was thriving then, and lots of people came to our door. Their numbers quickly grew too great for our small house.

The time came for a change. In September 1973, fifteen of us, including Linda, J. J., and twelve others, took an eleven-month trip through Europe, North Africa, and Russia. When we returned, we moved into a six-bedroom house on twelve acres in Fairfax County, Virginia. It was synchronicity—the place came exactly the way we needed it and when we needed it. For three years it provided the model of what we wanted for the rest of our personal and professional lives. Twenty of us—J. J., another doctor, my brother, Linda's brother, a lawyer, a teacher, a farmer, some builders, Linda, and I—lived and worked together. As well as practicing free medicine, we focused on developing ways of creating intimacy and openness, something we had explored on our trip abroad. Linda and I were married there, and our first son, Zag, was delivered at home with all our friends in attendance.

The beautiful setting and the space were very important, because nature is a major part of our medicine. Two acres were set aside for animal and plant gardens. We built a tree house and an outdoor stage and produced all kinds of shows. We took quiet walks in the evening and had total privacy to do whatever we wanted. We held craft fairs, made movies, and explored play in many forms.

Every month, between a hundred and a thousand people came through the house, some for an hour, some for many days. We had anywhere from one to fifty overnight guests *every night*. They came because they'd heard we offered alternative therapies, didn't charge for our services, and had fun. We were a family practice taking care of every medical condition from birth to death. We saw people who wanted to kill themselves, who were fighting with loved ones, or who were having the kinds of problems hotlines handle. They came for every kind of reason, from school physicals to help with dying. Some said they came because of a particular problem, but when they started to leave, they'd say, "By the way, I . . ." and *that* would be the reason they came. Some of them, if asked today, would say, "Oh, I never was a patient." Regardless of how they presented themselves, I tried to have a friendship with almost every person who came by. We took walks in the woods together, watched sunsets, washed dishes, worked in the garden. These one-to-one encounters were the most important part of my experiment in healing.

One person who came as a patient still lives with us today. Gareth Branwyn is my ideal patient: a person who comes for medical care and with whom I form a friendship during the very first encounter. Gareth came to us in 1976 because of a profound form of arthritis that he'd had since the age of thirteen. Norman Cousins had a much milder form of the same condition, ankylosing spondylitis. Gareth was young—nineteen or so—and was very depressed about his arthritis. But we helped him see a bigger picture. Today, when you speak to Gareth, he has a lot more to talk about than his arthritis. He stayed with us for a week or ten days, and that sealed our lifetime together as friends.

People came for nonmedical reasons as well, such as the appeal of communal living. And they came to us for fun. One day a teacher who lived in the neighborhood and had heard about us dropped in. It was his birthday and he was lonely and depressed about having to be by himself. So he went out and bought a cake, drove over to our house, and said, "I heard you are nice people and I wanted somebody to have a birthday with." Everyone stopped what they were doing and we had a birthday party. It was great fun. We never saw him again, but I'm sure he still remembers that day as fondly as I do.

Many visitors who shared activities with us came back later when they were ill. The fact that we had started a relationship earlier had a positive impact, I'm sure. In this sense, everybody was a patient: visitors, friends, staff. In addition, we were all building relationships that would protect us against disasters like malpractice suits. How can you sue somebody you really like?

When you operate a wild extravaganza of activity day after day, some strains naturally develop among people. We took great care to practice preventive medicine in our interpersonal relationships. Never having received lessons on how to get along with a spouse or friends, much less a community, we proceeded by the seat of our pants.

Friendship was the number one key to our success. We loved one another, and love forgives a lot. In a marriage, the partners compromise; this was a big marriage. So if one person is messy and one is neat, in a good marriage the neat person becomes messier, and the messy person gets neater. And that's pretty much what happened. The super-neat people—and I'm one of them—did more than their share of work in the clean/messy department. The messy people did more work in some other department. In a community that loves one another, forgiveness and compromise become a part of life. We tried to accept one another. We even made it part of the humor.

We had started living communally like Babes in Toyland: naive, innocent, ignorant. We had no idea that the big discussions would be around quiet versus noise, neatness versus messiness, and so on. At times when we felt someone was being unfair, we would bring it up and talk about it in a constructive spirit. Fortunately, we were an extremely open group of people, but not everybody was a verbal communicator like me. Some communicate with words, others with deeds. So we had to experiment with ways of resolving conflicts, sometimes by having long discussions and sometimes by just saying "yes." In a way, being open was part of the therapy; not everyone was open, but we were all open to the extent that we were able.

The other key to our success was fun. From the start it was obvious that we had to have fun or the staff would have left in a week. (For example, one day everybody surprised me with a bathtub full of oiled noodles. I squished around in it while they performed the "Noodleloni Ballet.") Not only was fun a glue for our community, it had overwhelmingly beneficial effects on our patients, who needed fewer pain medications. With a mixture of compassion and humor, we ran a Monty Python medical facility. We did a huge amount of celebrating and gave special birthday parties for one another. Guests brought added wealth as they shared their interests. We held dances two or even three nights a week. We did stage productions of all kinds and produced children's fairy tales. We filmed about seventy hours of

Super-8 movies documenting our fun: cooking meals, tending the garden, playing in the mud, playing with our children, seeing patients.

People often ask, "How did you earn a living if you weren't charging your patients?" The answer, at first, was that we lived communally to keep expenses low and held part-time jobs. At Danville Street we were quite poor; each person had to contribute $19 a month for rent. We worked at various part-time jobs to pay for food and medical supplies. By the third year, when we lived at West Ox Road, I worked as a file clerk for $3.25 an hour at Planning Research Corporation in Arlington. After nine months, I worked for a medical nutritionist and did muscle biopsies. The pay was good—I earned $20,000 to $30,000 a year for the next two years by working only twelve hours a week.

Meanwhile, J. J. worked nights at St. Elizabeth's emergency room doing pre-admission physical evaluations, a job I took later when he quit. After a psychiatrist certified that newly admitted patients were mentally ill, I would take a medical history to certify whether they needed immediate medical attention. I probably admitted 6,000 to 8,000 people. Often I spent an hour or more with each patient, telling many who seemed open to it that I felt they could live mentally healthier lives. My shift was four nights in a row, sixteen hours a night. Then I'd be off for ten days. By working the equivalent of about eight days a month, I earned $45,000 to $50,000 a year. It was a good job. It provided a wealth of experience, a chance to help people in anguish, a lot of extra money, and spare time to explore other interests. I worked at St. Elizabeth's for eight years, from 1978 to 1986.

We also were sustained by gifts from friends. People would come by with all the makings for dinner and cook it for us. We received food, clothing, kitchenware, dishes, books, sheet music, garden equipment, used vehicles, furniture, even animals. A herd of half a dozen goats—crosses between Nubians and LaManchas—was probably our most exotic gift.

Our goat-herding venture began at The Rocks, an eighty-acre farm in Jefferson County near Charlestown, West Virginia, where we moved in 1977. The Rocks was an idyllic setting on a half-mile front along the Shenandoah River; it was also the first property our commune had ever owned. It cost us $240,000, which was owner-mortgaged on a $40,000 down payment. It was very difficult for a commune to get a commercial bank loan.

Linda and I were goatherds for the next five years. At the outset, we had no idea how to raise goats. We learned by making mistakes, talking to friends who could teach us, and reading books and magazines. As the herd increased to two dozen, we learned how to milk goats and make goat cheese. We became familiar with their veterinary needs and lanced many abscesses, which are a recurrent problem with goats. We had trouble keeping the goats confined; they could jump over a six-foot fence and sometimes escaped in the middle of the night. Linda and I shared the adventures of chasing them, but I had the job of slaughtering and skinning the males. We sold goat milk, cheese, hides, and sometimes the entire goat, as goat meat is a delicacy for many African peoples.

At The Rocks our patient load peaked; people from forty states and eighteen countries visited us. Despite our idyllic setting and dedication to providing free medical care, the support staff slowly showed signs of burnout. For years our home had been invaded by hordes of people. We worked outside jobs so that we could practice free health care; in a sense not only did we not charge money, we *paid* to see patients. And we didn't have beds for most of them. They were camped on the floors, in our bedrooms, in our hallways. It was chaotic. Not having a bedroom, not having privacy, not having enough beds for the patients proved an incredible strain. Most people wouldn't have lasted a month under these circumstances, but my friends lasted eight years.

Through all those years I had talked about how we would have a hospital, but we weren't getting any closer to having one. These staff members had lasted all those years through sheer fun, friendship, and the love of caring for others, but they burned out from not seeing the venture go anywhere. They wanted to cut back on giving health care and bring back some order into their lives. I never sensed any burnout in myself, and I think J. J. experienced very little, but I realized how hard it was for others. I could have fought them to keep our facility going, but the fight wasn't in me. Reluctantly, I decided that a split-up was necessary to accommodate those who needed to cut back and those who needed to move forward.

Leaving The Rocks was the saddest time of my life but a very important event. In hindsight, it was necessary to give the others a break from the project and for the rest of us to demonstrate that we were very serious about it. We were going to go on. J. J. stayed behind at The Rocks for a year and a half to take care of patients who were still coming there for health care. Then he went to India on a spiritual quest for a year and a half before returning.

The Rocks still functions as a commune, with the same people. We still are friends. With each one of those people I go back twenty years or more, and that's a long friendship to have. Most people have only one or two twenty-year friendships in their lifetimes, if that. Whenever I visit The Rocks, I have fifteen of those friendships already in place.

Linda and I moved nearer to D.C. to reorganize our efforts and devote more time to fund-raising. We rented a house on Centreville Road in Herndon, Virginia, with 100 acres—more than enough space to tend our herd of goats. In February 1980 a guest, not knowing that linseed oil spontaneously combusts in confined areas, put some linseed oil–soaked rags in the trash. A fire started in the night. Linda and Zag were almost burned to death in the confusion. While they stayed at Linda's parents' house, recovering from the fire, I lived in the burned house. One day while I was doing my best to keep myself, the goats, and everything else afloat, the phone rang. A friend read me an ad from a local newspaper in Pocahontas County, West Virginia, describing 310 acres of land for sale. We had been looking for land for many years and had asked a network of people to keep a lookout for us.

Despite a blizzard raging from D.C. to West Virginia, the instant I heard the description I called a friend who owned a four-wheel drive and said, "Frank, I could use a positive thought. Why don't you drive me to look at this land in West Virginia. This could be our land." We drove for six hours through the blizzard, the last twenty-eight miles through a scenic fairyland. We met the real estate agent and walked among the snow-covered trees and mountainsides. I sat on a rock behind a waterfall, looking out through a sparkling veil at the surrounding scenery. Everything cried out, "This is us!" The price was right—$67,000—so I told the agent, "I'll take it!"

In a way, finding the property was like reaching the Promised Land. It injected a renewed sense of purpose. Our fund-raising efforts, just barely begun, shifted into high gear. We decided to move another step closer to D.C. and in 1981 rented a tiny house on Fillmore Street in Arlington, Virginia. Gareth Branwyn and his wife, Pam Bricker, moved in with Linda, Zag, and me. They had lived at the Twin Oaks community, and Gareth decided to move closer to offer us his organizing, publishing, and philosophical skills. Ever since coming to us as a patient five years earlier, Gareth had been an active volunteer because we had helped him so much. He now could offer his intelligence and skills on a full-time basis.

In a sense, we were entering the second of three phases for the Gesundheit Institute. In phase one, the pilot project, people came to us in our home for help. During phase two, which I call fun(d)-raising, we have been reaching out to the world for help. In the course of this adventure, I have met many of the people I've been curious about in the medical and healing professions, in the performing arts, in building and architecture, and in all walks of life. And I'm meeting them not only for fund-raising but for global connectedness. The third phase will be the realization of our dream, building our hospital in West Virginia, where once again the world will come to our door.

7 • The Dream Defined

We are a company of friends, of givers and receivers, of doctors and patients.

Gesundheit Institute is a model health care facility based on a pilot project and on years of subsequent study. The time for such a model is long overdue. Extensive publicity, traveling, and networking have enlisted enough volunteers to staff five such free hospitals, if they existed. All these people need now is a context in which to serve.

Because we believe that health is everything that touches a person in a positive way, Gesundheit is designed as a total community. Our goals are to:

• Transform the traditional distinction between doctor and patient by creating an acute-care facility that is both a forty-bed hospital for patients and a home for forty full-time caregivers and their families

• Care for our caregivers by trying to operate a burnout-free facility

• Offer a wide choice of allopathic and alternative healing techniques: faith healing, acupuncture, homeopathy, internal medicine, surgery

130

• Integrate medical care with agriculture, natural surroundings, arts and crafts, performing arts, recreation, education, social services, friendship, and fun

• Help patients benefit from the healing power of intimacy and mutual interdependence

• Teach patients about preventive health care and personal responsibility for their health

• Create a model that will revitalize our decaying rural health care system

• Be a teaching institution for health care professionals, from medical and nursing students to hospital administrators

• Provide thirty beds for short-term volunteers and professionals attending training sessions

• Show that an individual is not a lone organism but part of a family, community, and world, all of which are in need of assistance and love

• Maximize the health and happiness of all who are at Gesundheit, both those needing care and those providing it

• Operate out of deep concern for the quality of people's lives in a world dominated by the values inherent in power and greed

• Create an environment of hope and the possibility of change

We define "health" as happy, vibrant, maximum well-being. It is focused on the patient's relationships to himself or herself and to nutrition, exercise, faith, family, friends, hobbies, nature, wonder, curiosity, creativity, service, community, and peace.

We will try to create an experience that enables every person who comes for help—however lonely, sad, anxious, angry, or pained—to find respite and get close enough to nature, fun, or God to reach toward his or her dreams. Doctor (giver) and patient (receiver) will work side by side to accomplish all the tasks at hand. Each individual will serve as a custodian for the whole facility. We will assemble a staff so diverse that all patients can find at least one person who loves and understands them. We will nurture deep friendships between health givers and receivers.

Wonder and curiosity will be the air we breathe. Creativity will be encouraged in the staff and in all who visit us. Patients will be urged to express themselves in whatever art form they choose. They will have opportunities to explore on their own and with others. Everybody will enjoy countless opportunities to find ways to help other people.

In summary, we will extend our happy, funny, loving, cooperative, creative community—owned by no one, served by all—to benefit people everywhere. As it has done in the past, this atmosphere will enhance health and relieve suffering in a unique way. The practice of medicine will become a joy in such surroundings.

Our Ethics

The issue of medical ethics is complex, but there are issues around which we must formulate policy and communicate it. When faced with a population as diverse as that of the United States, where all kinds of contradictory beliefs coexist and individual choice is sacrosanct, no facility can truly represent that population if it dictates one approach or one set of beliefs. Much time must be spent understanding and respecting the beliefs of each person who comes to us.

We believe that the facility belongs to our patients. Therefore, we have formulated very little group policy on morality beyond the necessity of functioning for the common good. For the most part, we will address issues of availability. We want to care for all people equally, without preferential treatment, whether or not the patient has helped create or maintain the facility. We will strive to give the broadest possible care, including standard pharmaceutical and surgical approaches and alternative forms of care. We hope that whoever comes will have an opportunity to explore all kinds of therapies in a safe, supportive environment. The staff will accept all kinds of practitioners and respect their expertise. When two or more systems collide, they will be prepared to work through conflict with a dialogue in which everybody can participate. Above all, no health care professional will have to implement a treatment that he or she does not support.

Ultimately, the choice of therapy will be the patient's. We will strive for intimacy so that individual choices grow out of a whole-system analysis. We have seen miracles and disasters in all methods of care. One can never promise a given result with any treatment. Each is a gamble. As a result, we feel morally obligated to promote personal responsibility for a healthy lifestyle to lessen the need for imperfect choices.

One focus will be mutual interdependence. We are a company of friends, of givers and receivers, of doctors and patients. Everybody needs one another, so we will give all staff equal labor and respect. We will share in maintaining the facility, serving as doctor, maid, farmer, or artist—all in one. No duty will be valued more than another. Instead, we will function as one organism, with all parts contributing to a vibrant whole. We will rely on this interdependence as a major healing force, both individually and globally in our interface with the world. We support total nuclear disarmament and preservation of the troubled environment. These, we feel, are the most pressing moral issues facing health care professionals and society today.

On some very complex moral issues we will withhold judgment. We do not believe these controversial subjects can be covered by blanket morality without interfering with our patients' sovereignty and right to choose. Abortion is such an issue. We do not condone abortion as a form of birth control and acknowledge that this procedure can cause profound trauma, but we feel obligated to respect the choice of every woman involved. We will make a great effort to provide sound education about sex and birth control. If a woman chooses to have an abortion, we will provide it and hope that our environment will help her readjust to life afterward. We also will be supportive of women who wish to have their babies and either keep them or give them up for adoption. We hope to offer the option of finding people who will adopt the child of a woman who does not want an abortion.

Death with dignity is a vital issue. We hope that individuals and their families will develop the deep intimacy needed to clarify how they would like to be treated if, as the result of illness or accident, they are unable to communicate their wishes about resuscitation or life support systems. We will encourage our patients to draft a living will. Then we will try to follow the best route, preferably one already discussed with family members.

A final moral issue is malpractice insurance. We recognize that all health care professionals are fallible and may make mistakes throughout their careers; we also feel strongly that friendship, open communication, and trust constitute the best prevention against being sued for malpractice. At Gesundheit, we cannot and will not practice in fear and mistrust. We intend to practice as a diversified and highly qualified group, drawing on one another's expertise and advice with the goal of never bringing harm to another person. We will use a rigorous selection system to ensure competence among all our practitioners and caregivers. All of us will care with all our ability and will put the patient's well-being first.

As long as the science of medicine is imperfect, it is wrong to expect infallibility. If a patient feels dissatisfied with his or her care, we want to know immediately. We will investigate, evaluate, and if necessary dismiss any staff member who has been negligent. We will always make every attempt to correct the consequences of any mistake.

Our Staff

The most difficult task at Gesundheit is helping staff and patients become—and stay—healthy and happy. Obviously, these attributes first must be established in the staff. One reason for Gesundheit's unique design is to create a burnout-free environment. If we operate a hospital where staff members are always burned out, patients are going to be burned out too. We hope that if staff members do leave, the reason will be that Gesundheit was not the right place for them, but my deepest desire is for a staff that will never leave.

Some individuals, no matter how they practice medicine and deliver health care, are going to suffer burnout just because of their personalities or their approaches to life. I don't want burned out professionals on the staff. I want professionals who hunger to work with people, who will be fulfilled and energized by serving others and by living in the creative, outgoing, exciting environment that Gesundheit offers. Naturally anyone who feels the need for a break from the work should take one, but this should be done in an atmosphere of commitment.

By the time we open, I will have enlisted several family doctors, a general surgeon, obstetrician-gynecologist, pediatrician, ophthalmologist, psychiatrist, dentist, midwife, chiropractor, homeopath, acupuncturist, naturopath, and nurses. Many of the staff will offer massage therapy and meditation sessions. Ideally, each member of our team will have many talents, so that some expertise will overlap.

Our support staff will include farmers, mechanics, builders, artists, craftspersons, and a lawyer—both for Gesundheit and for patients who need legal advice. We want two teachers for children—ours, sick kids, and family members of patients. All community members, including spouses or partners, will be part of our staff and will contribute their diverse talents.

The labor for most of our efforts will continue to be volunteer, but if we cannot find volunteers for specific tasks, we will hire the needed person. We will feed and house our workers, offering them free room and delicious food in a beautiful setting, wonderful friends, hard work, good fun, and an important role in creating a model health community.

We will have thirty beds for people who help us for a limited time (I am asking for a minimum two-year commitment); they will range from physicians and carpenters to wandering minstrels and bird-watchers. These people will bring a great wealth of skills and interests.

When we began the pilot project, our staff members were in their twenties. Now we are mostly in our thirties and forties. I hope to have people of all ages on our staff. Grandmothers and grandfathers often serve a function just by being their old, wise selves. In a friendly and joyous situation, old people can add a wonderful edge to all of the other ages. They contribute wisdom and knowledge; most of all, they embody a positive accumulation of experience.

Our staff should be happy, loving, funny, cooperative, creative, and able to generate self-esteem and positive thinking in themselves and others. By their style of living, the staff should set an example of good relationships for patients. I want staff members who willingly give up huge amounts of private time in a facility where at least one caregiver is always available to work with each patient and can accept constant interruptions. If staff members are to tackle gigantic social problems, they must be prepared to devote their lives to it. They must see the project not only as a hospital operating in West Virginia, but as community and world peace. Staffers must be in love with the dream.

A Patient's Stay at Gesundheit

As a doctor, I experience hospitals as gloomy places. Seldom do you see hospital staff members bounding down the halls, thrilled by the privilege and joy of helping others. Patients in most hospitals experience nightmares of fear and impersonal treatment. The atmosphere at Gesundheit Institute will be upbeat and unlike other modern medical facilities. Many of our patients will be unhappy when they arrive, suffering not only from physical ailments but from the loneliness and low self-esteem that are components of many illnesses. If only physicians could turn on a switch that would make patients' lives happy, health would be greatly improved. But there is no such switch or pill. Patients must find happiness for themselves. What we *can* offer—and what few other medical facilities offer—is fertile ground for people in pain to discover happiness.

The concept of treating the whole person, and of viewing people as more than their diseases, implies a huge amount of psychological and spiritual work. That is why Gesundheit integrates healing with agriculture, recreation, performing arts, arts and crafts, and living together in community.

We recognize that each person is unique, and we will tailor the visit to his or her needs. No two visits will be alike. For an example of what a visit might be like, picture yourself as a man, thirty-seven years old, married with two children. You have just been diagnosed as having ulcers, a very common disorder. Your doctor calls and gives us the full report; then we speak to you by telephone. We invite you to visit, with your family, for a week or ten days. You are encouraged to bring musical instruments, fishing gear, books, and other leisure-time items.

If you come by car, before you reach us, you will have journeyed through the beautiful West Virginia hills. Turning into the 310 acres of Gesundheit, you will see in the distance the main facility: a wood, stone, and concrete structure rising up at the foot of a mountain. Driving toward this facility, you will pass the woodworking shop and crafts buildings on the left and, beyond that, food and flower gardens. The natural beauty will touch you before you ever reach the building.

The main entrance will connect with a long overhead footbridge spanning the roadway like a gate. At the other end of the bridge, you may notice a meditation area amid the crops. A staff member will greet you in the central lounge area, a four-story space rising to a sunlit glass dome. After a brief tour, your host will check you in and tell your children and spouse about that day's activities. For the children, exploration and play are available; for your spouse, the same on an adult level.

Meanwhile, you will meet with the therapist of your choice—whether in allopathic medicine, homeopathy, acupuncture, or some other discipline. You will learn that you can try several kinds of therapeutic methods throughout your visit and even can observe various healers in action beforehand.

First, however, you will participate in an extended two- to four-hour interview as part of a complete medical and social history and physical exam. This interview will lay a foundation for openness and an all-important friendship with your therapist. You will fully explore your reasons for coming to Gesundheit Institute and what you hope to gain from the visit. You will be asked about all areas of stress in your life: family, work, and personal. The therapist will discuss which tests and studies need to be done and will outline a treatment plan that addresses both your ulcers and the quality of your life in general.

You will be advised to try gentle, inexpensive treatments first to see whether they solve the problem. Exercise, diet, recreation, and work will be part of your therapy. Many stress-reducing activities will be available each day, including meditation, massage, nature walks, theater, crafts, and play.

During this time, your spouse will meet with a staff member to express his or her feelings and needs. With your permission, we may even call upon other family members or friends for their perspectives. In this way, your spouse, children, and friends will be enlisted into a health team for you and for one another.

Throughout your stay, we will observe your response not only to your family but to others at the facility. Since all staff and patients at Gesundheit interact, we will note the feelings of all who come in contact with you about your response to recreation and work. Any suggestions or insights that may arise will be brought to the attention of your primary caregiver, who will decide whether they should be implemented in your basic care plan.

Although spontaneity is important at Gesundheit, some daily routines will be established. Early mornings may be spent in exercise and meditation. Breakfast will provide an informal time for discussing the day's activities with the staff and other patients and deciding who will do what. You will then set out on your appointed tasks: therapy, work, recreation, or all three. Dinner will be a major gathering time when everybody will eat together and share the day's events.

Nighttime activities may include discussions and workshops on various topics, socializing, dancing, games, music, or being alone.

A primary reason our community is healing is that we all work in the gardens, harvest, cook food, serve food, and clean up afterward. In most families, Mom does that. We're not anybody's mother. We're trying to be doctors for a society that is disturbed and beset by boredom, loneliness, and greed. If society is the patient, then we need medications that will help improve a sick society. One of the great medications for a sick society is interdependence, or people feeling "at one" with society and one another. This means that both permanent residents and guests will work to the extent of their physical abilities. Everybody who comes to Gesundheit will be assigned to a cooking team and a clean-up team. Other tasks will involve farming and gardening activities, maintenance, arts and crafts, cottage industries, child care, and education.

Our entire concept of community and interdependence requires that patients become emotionally *independent*. In exposing you to the experience of community, we also will help make you *interdependent*, because we believe this will be beneficial to your health. For example, we will explore how your interests can be integrated with those of the staff and other guests to promote interdependence and friendship. People who play chess will be matched. People who are artistic or skilled will be encouraged to do projects together. There is great medicine in helping others; people who are dependent or used to having others wait on them will be assigned to take care of a person with quadriplegia or someone who is dying. Since many men in our society don't have women friends, male patients may spend time with one of the women on our staff. You will be asked to share some skill or knowledge with the community, so that you will feel useful. You will have many possible paths to follow. If you are not open to wonder, curiosity, humor, love, or alternative healing systems, we'll try to put you in touch with the diverse environment at Gesundheit.

Part of everyone's therapy, we believe, is to explore responsibility to one's self and one's community and to help with the tasks of daily living. A patient afflicted by loneliness may join several medical students, a wandering musician, a cancer patient, several people suffering from so-called mental disorders, and children on a three- to four-day camping trip in the surrounding national forest. From such encounters will come interdependence, human bonding, creative living, appreciation of nature, and effective ways of dealing with stress.

When a person is unable or unwilling to do his or her share, it shows up in loneliness, selfishness, and sometimes even a health problem. Consider the thousands of people who talk about how great it feels to be able to work. And consider how horrible they feel when they're in a conventional hospital and not taking part in the action. How many people who have been hospitalized have ever felt any connectedness to the place? How many say, "I just had a fabulous day in the hospital! Sorry to go! Wish I were sicker!"? At Gesundheit, patients are going to say such things routinely.

By the end of your visit, we hope that you, the staff, and others at our facility will have become friends. We will encourage frequent follow-up letters and phone calls, and maybe a weekend camping trip to Gesundheit each year for a check-up and refresher "course." If we know of appropriate people in your hometown, we will put you in touch, hoping that friends of Gesundheit will become friends of one another.

What We'd Like to Know About Patients

Initial interviews with patients last three to four hours and explore not only their health needs but everything about them. The following synopsis gives an idea of the detailed information we seek from patients in attempting to know them and to assess their health needs. Ideally, we would like each person in our care to write (in readable form) a detailed history of his or her life from a health perspective, and include the following:

1. Any facts pertaining to birth or the first years of life

2. History of immunizations up to the present

3. Hospitalizations, with dates and details

4. All remembered illnesses, with current perspectives on each

5. Drug-taking history, legal and illegal, including perceptions of drugs; include tobacco, caffeine, sugar, alcohol, etc.

6. History of spiritual perspectives, including past influences and current attitudes

7. History of love life with present perspectives and how they evolved, with comments on each of the following in detail: parental love, romantic love, sexual love, love of life, self love, any other

8. History of major disappointments, past and present, including solutions found, and perceptions of other people's disappointments

9. History of life highlights, including significant teachers (either formal education or on one's own). List skills of any sort gleaned from these high points: how they were acquired, appreciated, and shared with others. Also include highlights derived from books, movies, music, intellectual pursuits, etc.

10. A detailed family tree with health and other perspectives on each branch

11. Thoughts on what growing up was like, descriptions of homes, schools, neighborhoods, best friends, pets, travel, clubs, dates, cars, motorcycles, hobbies, and whatever else seems significant

12. History of diet, past and present, including present practices, perspectives, and theories about nutrition

13. Dreams for the future

14. Comments on success/failure, right/wrong, winning/losing, happiness/unhappiness as they relate to dealings with parents, children, jobs, life, lifestyle, community, country, spiritual values, friends, enemies

15. Perspectives on present state of body: strength, stamina, and joint flexibility; exercise habits; use of baths, oils, saunas, massage, and herbs; bowel and urine habits; condition of eyesight, hearing, and other sensory organs

16. Perspectives on death (one's own and others), including personal experiences with death

17. Perspectives on mental illness, in oneself and in others; is there such a thing as mental illness?

18. Ways to expand health consciousness, including how to use resources to help give health to yourself and others

19. Other details about health that this list has stimulated

If you hear us repeatedly asking for this report, we're just eager to optimize each patient's health care. We will also include baseline physical examination results in each patient's records—blood pressure, heart tracing, urinalysis, blood work, acupuncture diagnosis—all for free. There are thousands of effective ways to build health. Let's collect as many as possible.

You are a Gesundheit patient for life. After you leave, send a yearly updated addendum. We need this information to understand how to practice preventive care with each patient and to share the resulting insights about health with others. We have made a great time commitment to our patients' health; please return the commitment in this report.

Remember, no report is too long. Grant us permission to show other staff members and patients this report; we all can be great teachers of ourselves.

8 · Gareth's Story

Gareth Branwyn

We watched a beautiful orange sunset in silence, and Patch turned to me and said, "Do you have arthritis while you're watching this?"

When I was twelve years old, I incurred what appeared to be a sports injury. I sprained a toe and it wouldn't heal. My toe was swollen and sore for months, but the doctors could find no cause or cure. That summer I had a night job washing floors at J. C. Penney. When my knees started swelling up, the doctors said the cause was my being on my knees so much.

Then, at the age of thirteen, I woke up one morning with an intense pain in my hip. I couldn't get out of bed. My mother took me to the doctor, who examined me, took X-rays, and concluded: "It's just growing pains. Gareth is very tall and he's growing too fast. Try these pain pills and muscle relaxants, and he'll be fine."

It went on like that for years. More doctors, more pills, more pain. They decided that I had juvenile rheumatoid arthritis, but they were wrong. It was years before I was correctly diagnosed. When I was seventeen I moved to the Twin Oaks community in Louisa, Virginia. After a year or so, the pain started getting worse. When my back became involved, I was really frightened.

The Twin Oaks community sent me to the nearby University of Virginia Medical Center in Charlottesville. The doctors there tested me and discovered that I had ankylosing spondylitis, a form of arthritis that destroys the spine and all the major joints of the body— "the fight to remain upright," as one patient education pamphlet melodramatically stated. I was eighteen years old and had an incurable disease that might kill me.

One of the health counselors at Twin Oaks, Vince Zager, was interested in alternative healing. He and I began exploring different therapies one by one. Whenever we heard about a new system, we'd inquire about the arthritis remedy and how long it would take to get results. Usually these therapies were supposed to bring about at least a glimmer of improvement in one to three months. For that amount of time, I would follow the regimen almost to the letter. If I saw no change at all, I would move on to the next thing. Whenever any healing method seemed moderately promising, we would travel to the place where it was offered. Twin Oaks paid for legitimate health bills, which included those for unconventional therapies. I could not have afforded them on my own.

I tried wheat grass therapy (blended wheat grass juice three times daily), Bach flower remedies (tinctures made from plants that are supposed to have healing power), herbal therapy (based on various kinds of herbal teas that tasted like swamp water), peach pits, visualization, vibrations, crystals, and other New Age therapies. Once I was supposed to put a pillow on the floor and imagine it was the person who was the greatest hindrance to my development. I kicked and punched and yelled at the pillow, then got back in bed, hugged it, and told it I forgave it, visualizing the person the entire time. I did this for weeks. Every morning when I got up, everyone who lived in my building at Twin Oaks would hear me saying, "You bitch. You destroyed my life," and ten minutes later, "I love you. I forgive you."

All these therapies placed tremendous emphasis on following the regimen exactly. For example, a naturopathic doctor prescribed a treatment plan for three months. When I returned and reported no results, he asked, "Did you follow it to the letter?" I said, "Yes, absolutely." He said, "And there was *no time at all* when you veered from the plan?" I admitted to eating spaghetti, a forbidden food, once when I was in a hurry. He said, "Well, *no wonder* it didn't work!"

If I didn't have another program planned by the time I finished one of these therapies, I would revert to the regular Twin Oaks diet, which consisted of basic health foods. Sometimes I would eat whatever I wanted to during the interim. After two weeks of eating, drinking, and binging, I would feel great, because I had labored under all these strict regimens and felt guilty about not healing myself. During these interludes, I sank into irresponsibility and had the time of my life. My arthritis even felt better for a while. I started joking about how I was going to write a book about decadence as a cure for arthritis.

The bottom line, however, was that nothing helped. The last therapy I tried before meeting Patch Adams was a fourteen-day juice-and-water fast that was horrendous. I lost so much weight that I needed a thick pillow to sit on because my seat bones would hurt. By the end of the fast, I felt suicidal. I told friends that I would never be a productive person, I would never have a relationship with a woman, I had nothing to live for.

Around this time Vince, my counselor at Twin Oaks, met Dave Wember, a homeopathic physician who was working with Gesundheit Institute. They talked about whether homeopathy might help my arthritis. Vince also mentioned that I was very depressed. Dave told him that Patch worked very well with people who were depressed about having chronic diseases.

Vince urged me to call Patch, but I resisted because I had been through so many therapies by that point. But I let Vince call Patch for me while I listened on the other line. It was like something out of a Fellini movie. Patch sounded like a nice person, but his enthusiasm seemed a bit overbearing. Still, I called him back about fifteen minutes later. I remember two things about the conversation: He talked very loud—at one point I had to hold the phone away from my ear when he blasted "I *love* communes!" after learning that I lived in one—and, at the end of the conversation, he said, "We'll do everything we can to help you. But if help can't be had, you may have to get into the pain." I hung up the phone and felt really put off. All the New Age remedies I had tried emphasized doing everything possible to soften pain. I wondered, "What is he talking about?" Curiosity compelled me to find out.

A few weeks later, I traveled by bus to Fairfax, where I was met by Ozzy, the psychiatrist at Gesundheit. He was small and bubbly, with curly black hair, a salt-and-pepper beard, rainbow suspenders, and a tie-dyed T-shirt. I was trying to maintain an aura of "I'm-too-bummed-out-for-this," but inwardly I loved this guy immediately. He had a sense of humor like Woody Allen's.

He led me to a car containing two people he had just picked up from St. Elizabeth's Hospital in Washington. We headed for a farm off West Ox Road in Fairfax. The trip was wild. One of the passengers, a woman, showed me the suicide scars on her wrists while Ozzie chatted about his car, which was named Prince Valiant after the comic book character. I thought, "My God, I've landed in the loony bin!"

When we arrived at the farm, I saw, sitting in the parking lot, a bright red double-decker bus with a sign painted on the side: "We're all Bozos on this bus!" Circling the bus on a unicycle was a man with long hair, a huge mustache, surgical scrub pants, and a T-shirt that said, "Laugh your ass off!" featuring a little naked cartoon character whose butt was floating away because he was laughing so hard. I walked up to him, thinking "This *can't* be the doctor!" Ozzie said, "This is Patch!" While still riding the unicycle, he started conducting my health interview right then and there. He wasted no time whatsoever! After a while, he put the unicycle down and we went for a walk. It was a beautiful day and we toured the fourteen-acre farm, coming to a garden and sitting down next to a cone of teepee poles set up on a platform.

The interview disturbed me. Almost immediately, Patch asked me, "What's your passion in life? What turns you on? What motivates you? What excites you?" I said, "Not much. I like to read." He replied, "Isn't reading great? I *love* to read!!" I started telling him what I liked to read, but it was painfully apparent that he was one-upping me with his level of enthusiasm. I decided to ask about his favorite author. "Kazantzakis," he replied and began quoting from *Zorba the Greek:* "Life is trouble" and "A man needs a little madness, or else he never dares cut the rope and be free." He also quoted Zorba's line that the greatest tragedy is for a man to refuse a woman who invites him to her bed.

The whole point, of course, was passionate living. I read Kazantzakis later and understood this. But at the time, I was of two minds. I was really attracted to Patch's incredible personal power and obvious happiness with himself and his life. He also was warm and personable. As he continued to interview me out by the teepee, it grew late. We watched a beautiful orange sunset in silence, and Patch turned to me and said, "Do you have arthritis while you're watching this?" The question absolutely floored me. "No, come to think of it, I don't." "Do you have a girlfriend?" he asked. "Yes, sort of." "When you make love with her, do you have arthritis?" That was something I *had* noticed. Throughout all my attempts to control the pain of arthritis, any time I got turned on—alone or with my girlfriend—my hormones would kick in for half an hour or so, and I would feel no pain. Patch asked, "Are there any other times you don't feel pain?" "Sometimes when I'm at a party and dancing," I said, "my muscles relax and I'm free from pain."

So I had sunsets, sex, and dancing! Patch said, "All you need to do is indulge yourself in your passions and increase the amount of time your mind is not focused on your physical self." I had found a doctor who prescribed fun, relaxation, passion, and bliss!

He suggested that I read more and find other things to enjoy. It was the beginning of a lifestyle surrounded with friends, books, and pastimes that made me feel good. The more I dosed myself with things that were positive and pleasurable, the better I felt physically. I found myself literally drugging myself with endorphins (pain-relieving natural hormones) that were released every time I had a pleasant experience. Patch's question "How does it make you feel?" stuck in my mind. I never had asked myself that question. Now I focused on it and on how I *wanted* to feel. I learned to engineer situations that would make me feel better physically, mentally, spiritually, and emotionally and to leverage my situation, however hopeless it seemed, to its full advantage.

This experiment in self-healing continued for ten days. When my visit ended, I actually felt worse than when I'd arrived because I had spent the entire week partying, going to concerts, eating decadent food, and staying up late in passionate discussions about health, community, sanity, and rock and roll. I had completely violated the strict regimen that my health counselor at Twin Oaks had prescribed. But what I gained was more helpful than any other drug or treatment I had ever tried.

Before meeting Patch, I had always been in a me-against-the-world pain paradigm of life. I literally used to think, "Why does the universe oppose me like this?" When I first arrived at Twin Oaks, I was into Marxism, atheism, and anarchy. After meeting Patch, I became a much happier, more outgoing person. I even became one of the holiday events managers at Twin Oaks and helped produce plays, concerts, and all kinds of events. I discovered dancing.

I also discovered relationships. I had had only two relationships before meeting Patch, and they hadn't worked. During my visit I told Patch about a woman I wanted to date but didn't have the courage to approach. I say "date," but at Twin Oaks in the 1970s nobody really dated. When we asked somebody, "Do you want to have a date?" this meant that we met at the end of the evening, talked for an hour or so, and went to bed together. So a "date" basically was asking somebody to go to bed.

Patch said, "Why don't you ask her?" "I know she's not interested in me," I said. "I'm no catch. I have arthritis." Patch said, "Everyone has the right to fail. Why not accept, as the bottom line, that you're going to make a total ass of yourself. Anything you get beyond that will be gravy!"

I decided to try it. When I returned to Twin Oaks, I spent a week focusing on the thought that I was going to look like a fool. Then I asked the woman, "Do you want to have a date?" She said, "Sure, that would be great!" Just like that. What a huge change *that* made in my self-confidence and in just about everything!

After that, I started flirting mercilessly. I became really good at it. I flirted with women I wasn't even interested in, just for fun. It got to the point where I never asked a woman for a date who didn't accept, not because I was such an amazing catch but because my flirting told me, in advance, whether she would say "yes." These successes prepared me for the most important relationship of my life.

I had a crush on Pam before I ever met her. She was the editor of the Twin Oaks newsletter, which I had received while still living with my parents. I had taken a graphic arts class and was interested in writing, publishing, and Pam Bricker, because I liked the way she did the newsletter. When I moved to Twin Oaks and met her, she left a few days later. I didn't see her again for four years. When I temporarily left the community, she returned. When I came back to get my belongings, expecting to move to San Francisco, I fell in love with her and never left.

At first I hesitated to ask her for a date and spent several months flirting with her. She was in a relationship with my closest friend at the time, and I didn't want to interfere. But their relationship was not working out, and eventually she expressed her interest in me. One evening in October 1980 I saw her in the kitchen, and she asked, "Would you like to take a walk so we could talk for a few seconds." I sort of knew what was going to happen. As we walked, she said, "I think I've fallen in love with you." I remember saying, "I need to sit down!" I felt dizzy, I was so in love with her. We spent that night together, although it was nonsexual. Her boyfriend found out about it the next day and called off their relationship. Pammy and I have been together ever since.

My earlier relationships with women were nothing compared to this. The others were always tied in with my arthritis. Pammy has given me the greatest gift a person with an affliction could hope for: she never has focused on it. Yet she's always there when I need her. If I drop something in the next room, she comes in because she's heard it or has heard me say "Shit!" She picks it up, puts it back, and walks out. She's a super caregiver. In the years we've been together—we married in 1984—she rarely has mentioned my arthritis. Yet, it has to be a factor because she's a very physical person. We hardly ever go for walks or for rides in the car. She does my share of the housework. I don't have a cooking night anymore because I can't stand in one place for two hours at a time. Pammy does two cooking nights a week and never mentions it. If I start cleaning up after dinner, she'll come in and say, "Why don't you sit down? I'll do your clean-up." And I'll say, "Oh, no," because as long as I keep moving, I can manage.

Perhaps the greatest miracle of my life has been my son, Blake. At first I thought I could never be a father. Then, when Pammy became pregnant, I thought, "I'm never going to be able to pick up my child." I played tapes in my head saying I was going to fall short. Yet I picked up Blake until he was three years old. I have a horribly bad back, and it was painful, but I still was able to pick him up until he weighed about 35 pounds. Trying to lift anything else weighing 35 pounds would have been impossible, but the love and desire to be close to my son and hold him close overcame all the handicaps, all the pain, and I lifted him. Patch used to say, "God, Gareth, I can't believe you're still carrying him up and down the stairs!"

Back at the beginning, I wouldn't have had a child, let alone try to be a physical parent. I owe it all to what Patch taught me. We all need to dose ourselves with whatever is positive, upbeat, satisfying, and pleasurable—in my case, enjoying holding my son. This approach to life works so well that if doctors taught their patients even the smallest bit of it, the benefits would make them wonder why they ever thought they had a medical problem.

9 · Organizing Dreamers

Blair Voyvodic, M.D.

The entire purpose of a structure at Gesundheit is to support people's enthusiastic efforts to make the world a better, therefore healthier, place.

How does a group of well-meaning, idealistic, fun-loving caregivers get organized to make sure that everything gets taken care of? There is an organization to Gesundheit, and it's sufficiently unique to make it difficult to grasp. As a radical organization, we have worked at exploring the roots of how things function and have evolved creative models that are extremely different from traditional organizational structure.

The principles that guide our organization at Gesundheit are:

1. that our relationships are based on friendship;
2. that our motivation stems from the joy of service;
3. that fun is not only desirable, but a requirement in our work; and
4. that each person is responsible for his or her own delight.

The implication that our relationships are based on friendship isn't about us being friendly and chatty, and it certainly isn't about pretending to be friends. It means that we are interested in getting to know each other better, in learning what people's interests, thrills, and peeves are. It works best with a commitment to both honesty and openness. The better we get to know each other, the more obvious our interrelatedness is and the more naturally our spontaneous support flows.

This is in contrast to typical organizational structure that is based on positions of authority, most of which are task oriented. We do take on a variety of roles and tasks within the context of our primary relationship as friends. Our task-oriented roles are like different hats or costumes we put on; the person as friend remains the same. A key advantage of this is that it allows us to modify our roles creatively. It avoids the danger of letting people get stuck in positions that are not healthy for them.

The importance of friendships is highlighted if conflict arises in trying to make decisions. Between friends, conflict becomes an opportunity to get to know each other better by tracking down the underlying beliefs or understandings that the conflict is based on. It can be done with lots of heated debate, but the objective is to further understanding, not to "win." Our ideal is a consensus decision-making process because we believe it is better to keep working at deepening our friendships than it is to reach a quick decision that breeds resentment. This style works best when people are willing to dive into the complexities and convolutions of expanding intimacy, trusting that we will also reach effective decisions.

Part of the complexity for us is the huge personal investment that people make in Gesundheit. It is far more than a job. People work passionately because they feel their work makes a major difference in the world. There is an intimate link between the work and their most cherished dreams. For some people, Gesundheit is their lifework, dreams, friends, home, and sole source of income. Each level of involvement brings with it a personal stake in what goes on. Working through these intricacies to reach consensus is worthwhile for funda-mental decisions. For the vast majority of decisions, we rely on an extraordinary level of trust.

This starts with people trusting their own vision and being willing to act on it. You only need other people's permission to the extent that your actions create a demand on others. The more you ask for from Gesundheit, the bigger the burden on you to justify the demand. Demands are made in a variety of ways: taking people's time, attention, energy, enthusiasm, money, etc. Whatever the demand, the result is a shift from offering to be of service to asking to be served. On the other hand, to explore Gesundheit's resources as opportunities to dive into your own fantasy of making the world a better place, without creating demands on others, is to be of service in a way that is mind-bogglingly exciting. There is a won-derfully liberating aspect to being of service in this way. When you're not creating a demand on others, the only limitations are your own.

Like friendship, the joy of service also has major implications that extend far beyond being a simple, catchy slogan. It started out as a preventive to burnout but has become an art in itself. It means not relying on guilt or obligation, which are the more commonly used motivators. It also means that when something seems to need doing and no one is busting with enthusiams to do it, you have to reexamine the need for getting it done. If the need is strong enough, the choice then becomes either making it joyful by finding enough satisfaction in filling that need or creating alternatives for which there is enthusiasm. Sometimes this results in better solutions than you had initially. Almost always, this approach results in more satisfaction and a deepening of involvement.

There is a valuable lesson in this approach that can be applied to many situations that require working with change. Change that is deeply effective and positive presents a paradoxical challenge. On the one hand, there needs to be an appreciation and acceptance of how things are in the here and now. On the other hand, there needs to be an active intention to make things better. Nothing needs to change, and everything can improve. This is the way to avoid the two extrem-ist traps of activist's frustration or pessimistic complacency.

In day-to-day practices, these principles blend together as we notice each other's cheerfulness. Guilt and obligation quickly lead to grumpi-ness, in marked contrast to the goosebump-raising thrill of seeing someone working away inspired by the joy of service. As friends, we give each other support and feedback, which sometimes includes reminding each other that no task is worth sacrificing ourselves for. Not only will you not get appreciation for having sacrificed yourself, you may be reminded that your sacrifice has created more demand on others than if you had not made it.

This approach carries a significant requirement that each person be responsible for his or her own delight. It requires constant checking in with your own inspiration level. Good ways of doing that are noticing how much laughing you've been doing and honestly asking, "Am I having fun?" If you are truly having fun, then what you are doing is its own reward. You don't need to recuperate from healthy fun. It leaves you all set to dive into the next opportunity. Also, the more fun you're having with what you're doing, the easier it is for you to help other people have fun with you. It's contagious. If you're not having fun, if your enthusiasm is running low, you must be willing to recognize that refilling it is necessary for everyone's sake. Plugging away at something that you're not having fun with is a breeding ground for resentment. Even if you can avoid building up resentment, you start looking for rewards to justify your sacrifice, and rewards usually create demands on others. This requirement to infuse your work with fun can be very challenging at times, but it's well worth it.

As a diverse and radical organization we have our share of power dynamics. Since we don't have an authoritarian structure, there is no power granted by position or title. Power is gained by the consistency and effectiveness of the ways you contribute. As a person's contribution increases, the power of his or her influence increases. The main rule of thumb is: if you want something done, use the strength of that wanting to do it yourself joyfully. If this involves wanting other people to do something, it is your reponsibility to present your suggestion with enough enthusiam and inspiration that they will want to do it, either because they like the idea or out of support for you as a friend. This approach has been very frustrating for people who are accustomed to being in positions of power or who expect their suggestions to be carried out by "somebody." Rather than telling others what to do, at Gesundheit you are encouraged to trust your own capabilities and carry through on your own thinking.

Since Gesundheit is an ongoing experiment, our organization keeps evolving and growing. We are currently in the process of rethinking how we address issues of fairness and equality. Each person understands the commonly held vision in a unique way, and some people have clearer vision and deeper experience than others. Gesundheit is not an egalitarian community in that we are not all equally committed nor do we have equal experience. If our objective were to educate our staff, then restraining the more powerful folks to allow others to gain experience might be appropriate. But our primary aim is to be of service, and so we want everyone doing as much as they can possibly do—joyfully. Each person is encouraged to develop his or her own strengths but not at the expense of our collective work. In the long run, by ensuring that the collective work thrives, our community grows stronger, and we can create more opportunities for all members to gain enriching experience.

A final point on Gesundheit-style organization is leadership. There are many models for leadership. Our model is that leadership happens each time someone thinks about the group as a whole. What would be helpful for the whole group? What are the group's needs? When this perspective is balanced with consideration for the individuals in the group, the isolation of self-interest is eliminated. You can see more clearly what will be beneficial for the whole group as well as the individuals in it. Your effectiveness as a leader is strengthened the more you trust yourself as a leader and are willing to act with this perspective. This type of leadership does not rely on positions of power, it is available to everyone. In fact, the more people who take up leadership this way, the more smoothly and effectively everything works.

In summary, an analogy that I find useful is to see Gesundheit's organization as being like a flock of geese in flight (silly geese, of course). We are guided by a commonly appreciated need: for the birds it's to fly to warmth in the winter; for us it's to connect with others in being of service. Each bird is free to fly off independently but chooses to stay with the others because of the advantages. The work of the forward birds gives lift and cuts resistance to all that follow. Patch has been the lead bird throughout our history. Others of us are gaining strength with experience. Our goal is to become a group of powerful individuals led by a common vision, allowing Patch to be able to slip back to being one of the flock.

The entire purpose of a structure at Gesundheit is to support people's enthusiastic efforts to make the world a better, therefore healthier, place. I would like to extend an open invitation for anyone wanting to get involved to join us in our flight. Contact me, or any of us, to explore how you can do this.

Blair Voyvodic
RR 4
Killaloe, Ontario, K0J 2A0, Canada
e-mail: healing@web.net

10 · Building the Dream

Our Design

In considering a design for our facility, we have drawn on years of experience living successfully in group households. We have studied many philosophical constructs like Plato's *Republic* and Samuel Butler's *Erewhon*, and societies with a long history like the Shakers and the Amish. And we have been close to members of contemporary communities like Twin Oaks in Louisa, Virginia, and Findhorn in Scotland. These resources have helped us build and sustain community and learn how others have solved problems encountered by all groups. Many of our resources are listed in the Bibliography under "Community Living" (see page 198).

Over the last twenty years we also have explored the history of architecture, studying texts such as Walter Horn's and Ernest Born's *The Plan of St. Gall*, Christopher Alexander's *A Pattern Language*, and Ian McHarg's *Design With Nature*. These and other sources are listed in the Bibliography under "Building and Land Plan-

The atmosphere of the hospital is intended to avoid the indifference projected by so many facilities and to convey joy, enthusiasm, peace, caring, and openness.

154

ning" (see page 221). We have visited Chartres Cathedral, the Taj Mahal, and historical communities. Antonio Gaudí, who designed the Sagrada Familia in Barcelona, has been a strong influence. All the arts have exerted an influence on us, with their great power to inspire, relax, express, and teach. Because we consider them to be powerful therapeutic tools, we have designed into the facility the potential for theater, music, arts, crafts, and other forms of artistic expression for both staff and guests. We also wish to provide a setting for the artwork that many talented friends have donated or promised to us.

Concern for ecology has guided the land use and landscaping plans for our West Virginia land. Two of our members spent ten months learning about ecological management at the New Alchemy Institute in Falmouth, Massachussetts. This group explores sustainable farming, energy conservation, and appropriate technology to encourage a more environmentally sound relationship with nature.

In 1981, we brought our collective interests and design requirements to architects Dave Sellers and Bill Maclay of Warren, Vermont. We initially met them through a land plan they had prepared for the Renaissance Community in Turners Falls, Massachusetts. They had lived in community for many years and took our project to heart. These mavericks understood that what they were trying to do in architecture we were trying to do in medicine: set an example. Since 1981, they have been in continuous dialogue with us and have helped fantasize what we wanted Gesundheit to become. We have met numerous times and have visited the site together. Dave Sellers was on the land in July 1987 for an in-depth look at what we needed for the main facility. We spent a day walking imaginary patients through a week-long stay at the facility. Bill and Dave then designed the first of two buildings, an exquisitely crafted 6,000-square-foot craft and woodworking shop that is now complete. Bill has also completed a comprehensive land use and master plan that not only incorporates ecological and environmental data but identifies the spiritual qualities of the land's rich and varied features.

Dave, Daisy Rankin, and Mark deKay designed the main facility. They envisioned a hospital set back from the road with gardens, fields, and woods nearby. The atmosphere of the hospital is intended to avoid the indifference projected by so many facilities and to convey joy, enthusiasm, peace, caring, and openness.

The main entrance will be at one end of a long footbridge that spans the roadway like a gate. The clinic and emergency entrances will stand past the bridge under a canopy. This central forty-bed facility will house fully equipped, acute-care inpatient and outpatient services that can handle all aspects of rural medicine on a drop-in or scheduled basis. Emergency room, general surgery, X-ray, laboratory, pharmacy, ophthalmology, gynecology, acupuncture, dentistry, physical therapy, and many other specialties will be represented.

The central lounge will rise up four stories to a sunlit glass dome. This area will aid the passage of those waiting for or moving between treatment rooms. It will serve as a haven for people discussing various treatments with their therapists, relaxing before going to the dining room for lunch, or reading a book.

In the first-floor clinic a series of examining and consulting rooms, extending off the central communal area, will overlook the exceptionally beautiful landscape outside. These rooms will be supplemented by smaller areas for storage of medical records, supplies, and equipment.

Upstairs we will have forty patient beds, including five formal hospital-style beds with suction and oxygen. Since Gesundheit will try not to turn anybody away, this number reflects only the beds available, not necessarily the number of patients we can accommodate. When we don't have the needed space or equipment in the clinic, we will facilitate a patient's transfer to an appropriate facility such as the medical centers in Charlottesville, Virginia, or Charleston, West Virginia, or Lexington, Kentucky.

In addition, there will be rooms for each of our forty staff people and their families, large enough for sleep and some personal self-expression, plus thirty guest beds, arranged four to eight per room. Satellite rooms such as the birthing room will be reached by a bridge on the second floor. There a woman can give birth to her child with family and friends around her.

We will have special "fun" rooms where anyone can design and create an environment. Four other rooms will be dedicated to the elements—water, earth, wind, and fire. The shapes of these element rooms will be as unpredictable as the contents and ways in which they can be used.

There will also be a quiet 30,000-volume reference library with the usual horizontal shelves containing books, music, and videos, but with a twist: the spiral staircase joining book collections on the first floor to those on the second. Anyone can look down from the balcony at the bookworms below, but it will be up to the visitor to discover the secret trap doors, passageways, and swivel bookcases!

The dining hall will be the spiritual and social center of Gesundheit, for meals will be as much a part of the healing as any other facility activities. It will be capable of seating all residents, patients, and visitors. Three kitchens—regular, snack, and therapeutic—equipped with storage pantry, walk-in refrigerator, and freezer, will serve all meals, whether macrobiotic midnight snacks or communal dinners in fully equipped professional facilities. Since the entire Institute is cooperative, the evening's dietary selection may well be cooked by the same doctor who earlier tended to a patient's broken foot. All who are able will serve themselves. The dining hall will create a welcoming, homelike ambience and will be connected to the workshop, lake, and main common areas by gardens, pools, and paths.

Near the dining hall, a multipurpose hall with a 200- to 300-seat theater at one end will serve everyone at the facility, as well as the local community, with shows, concerts, lectures, and other events. The theater will include a professionally lit stage, where movies, aerobics, dance, and other events will take place. Resembling the Globe Theatre in design, it will have a floor gallery and two horseshoe-shaped balconies and will be double-faced so that performances can be enjoyed by audiences either outdoors, thanks to a movable stage wall, or indoors. A fireplace big enough to roast a mastodon, overhead skylights, and balconies are all part of the great hall.

Stimulating patients toward recovery plays a large part in our central building's design. We will have noisy areas for children, rambunctious adults, and the mentally and emotionally disturbed; game rooms and children's playrooms; craft rooms; and a two-story greenhouse. Special meditation areas and a quiet parlor with antiques and breakables will provide a different kind of environment.

Beyond the main facility, the master plan calls for many buildings and adaptations to landscape features throughout the land. Our 6,000-square-foot shop for heavy and fine woodworking and other crafts, completed in 1990, is the first of several buildings that will provide an expandable, pleasant place for people to work. These will include a ceramics pavilion, metals workshop, five-bay automobile repair garage with several hydraulic lifts, and two winterized bays. We have built a four-acre lake for swimming, fishing, canoeing, picnicking, cookouts, and other water-related activities.

Other projects we need to complete before opening are these:

• Renovate an existing old barn and possibly build a new one.

• Provide proper structures for about fifteen goats, a flock of sheep, and several hundred chickens. We will need barn space, chicken coops, and fencing. Work horses may be added as energy and money allow.

• Build a pole barn for tractor and farm machinery.

• Construct several small wooden bridges.

• Complete our roads.

• Landscape a flat area the size of a football field for games and helicopter evacuation.

• Build three large greenhouses in addition to the one attached to the main facility. The separate greenhouse will utilize wastes from graywater.

• Plant a wide variety of flower and food gardens, fruit and nut trees, and grape arbors.

• Provide access for the handicapped to the waterfall and other outdoor environments.

• Create a three-lagoon sewage system.

• Divert well and spring water sources to supply our needs.

• Clear several park-style paths up our mountain.

• Provide short- and long-term parking.

Additional projects we plan to complete after opening include access to the "rooms" in the cave behind the waterfall, retreat cabins, a temple for people of all faiths, and a simple log-cabin–style "great hall" for conferences and workshops. We hope to have, in addition, tree houses, gazebos, a maze with seating areas, and other outdoor recreational structures.

Individuals who have served two years as staff members and do not wish to live in the main facility will be allowed to build small houses or cabins in the village area. These living spaces will be small, simple, and partially built into the hillside. Designs will be approved by the governing body. There will be no vehicular access except for emergency and construction vehicles. The eventual maximum resident population will be less than 100 people.

Building on a Shoestring

To date, our building activity has involved housing our on-site staff of two to four people and a fluctuating number of volunteers and undertaking a variety of other projects as funds, materials, and available labor and skills allow. Many of these resources have come to us from people who have heard or taken part in our lectures, workshops, and shows.

The experiences of our summer volunteers typify what Gesundheit Institute is all about. A young woman from Germany wrote, "I have seen for the first time how positive life, people, attitudes, and even work can be." She was concerned about her return to dull, unrewarding work and wondered how to preserve what she had found in West Virginia. I wrote to her, "If you take positive, loving, fun attitudes *to* your work, you will have an impact *on* your work."

The first significant project was completed with help from many people, including ten volunteers from Service Civil International, a type of foreign peace corps that comes to the United States to help with worthy projects. Along with seven friends from the Twin Oaks community, neighbors, and friends of Gesundheit Institute, we transformed a small pond into a four-acre blue-green lake loaded with trout. A stream ran through our property, so we whacked weeds and cleared brush in preparation for excavating, dug out all the topsoil, moved it to the garden area, built a dock, excavated, hauled rocks for a spillway, and dammed up the creek. We even hauled in sand for a beach. It was the cheapest of the significant things we could do, and it provided a swimming hole for the local community.

The next major project was building the three-story, 6,500-square-foot workshop. This required money and took several summers to build. By 1984 we had completed the foundation and six-inch-thick, solid wood first-floor deck, giving us the best outdoor dance floor in West Virginia. By the summer of 1986 the framing was done, and a pyramid-shaped roof stood as a bold statement that Gesundheit

Institute would be built. Our crew of twenty or so, from many states, Canada, Italy, and Belgium, did the job in hard hats with rubber noses epoxied to the front. We have since built a barn, expanded an Appalachian-style shack that was on the property, and added two majestic yurts and other small buildings.

The new workshop was the setting for one of our greatest celebrations, the marriage of J. J. and Eva Bear in September 1987. J. J. had moved to the land in May 1983 to start building. The next year, Eva arrived, a single mother and an idealist dreamer. A friend had told her, "You ought to go and see this place," and she came and decided to stay. Three hundred friends came for the wedding, which was highlighted by two big dances in the workshop and a skit in which Eva's son, Josh, dressed as Cupid, was hoisted over the stage with a scaffolding rigging and shot arrows at the happy couple. It was a fabulous two-day celebration.

The next big project before we build the hospital will be a 10,000-square-foot bunkhouse that will house construction workers. Once our hospital is open, it will serve as a school and a place for patient and staff overflow. It also will be a place where we can start seeing patients on an outpatient basis until the hospital is completed. Our summer building projects have become annual extravaganzas, not only of hard work but of camping, hiking, swimming, fishing, hobbies, sports, mud pits, trough meals, rituals, and whatever else we collectively can think up.

Funding the Dream

For years I have tried to obtain foundation grants for the large sums of money needed for the hospital. When we received a few grants in the early 1980s, we prayed they would be a magnet for others, but we continued to submit grant proposals in vain. I have attributed this resistance of big-money organizations to the nature of our project, especially our refusal to accept fees or third-party reimbursement or to carry malpractice insurance. But on these issues we will not budge; they are major cancers of the health care system and must be excised. Foundations also may shy away because of our emphasis on humor. "You're not a serious project," they seem to say. So, unless the big funding sources have a change of heart—and we will continue to apply to them—our best hope is grass-roots funding.

At one point, in 1984, the foundation situation became so discouraging that Linda, Gareth and Pam, Louis and Cathy Fulwiler, and other friends decided to cheer me up with a surprise $50-a-plate birthday party for friends. They raised about $8,000, enough to start building on the land the following spring.

A terribly discouraging setback occurred in 1985 when one of our financial contributors offered to donate a large sum of money for the summer's building program *if* we could match it with an equal amount, with only fifteen days to raise the funds. After calling everyone we thought might donate, we were able to raise only half the amount needed and did not get the grant.

For the most part, however, we have been sustained by gifts from friends. We have received huge amounts of donated labor. Mechanics fixed my car. Carpenters helped us build. Lawyers did legal work. I sometimes opened a book and found a check in it. We received $30,000 to $40,000 worth of lab equipment. One person donated fifteen wheelchairs; a doctor in Maine gave us a used tractor and baler; the Twin Oaks commune donated printing equipment. As well as individual donations, some friends have used their contacts to raise money in their areas. Recently, a group in Santa Fe held a $100-a-plate fund-raiser that raised $7,000, and a woman in Wheeling, West Virginia, coordinated a year-long fund-raising drive that brought us $6,000. We have incorporated as a tax-exempt entity so that those who wish to make monetary donations can gain a tax advantage. The gifts have come in many forms but never in a debit/credit sense of reciprocating for services received. I prefer to think that people have given to us out of friendship or out of liking who we are.

Most of our donations are under $50 and have come from people of modest means, like the person who worked in a sock factory and sent a box of socks. An elderly woman in Iowa wrote: "I know you are a hospital so you'll need sheets; they are all clean." A woman in Haddonfield, New Jersey, wrote:

Dear Dr. Patch:

The enclosed check of $5 toward your hospital won't go very far, I know, but I send it with the humble prayer that God will somehow multiply it a thousand fold for you. And believe me when I say that it's the last $5 I have to my name. . . . I chose to give it to "Gesundheit" because I know the pain and humiliation of being turned away when I no longer had the money for *medical care. (I was undergoing treatment for a kidney infection and when I could no longer afford to continue treatment—well, that was just too bad.) Things got so desperate last winter that I wrote to six area clergymen begging for help—and you know, Patch, not one so much as answered my letter.*

So please hang in there, Patch—for the sake of those of us who have no one to turn to and no one to care. Without people like you, people like us literally have no choice but to crawl off in a culvert and die.

It's hard for people to give money for a dream. They have to be generous for their future. It's taken twenty years to earn $900,000. In total, we need $5 million for the forty-bed hospital, vegetable gardens, orchards, arts and crafts facilities, shops, and landscaping. Once the hospital is built, we will need $900,000 to $1.5 million a *year* to operate it. That means 10,000 people will have to send us an average of $100 a year. We have suggested that our friends donate one day of their annual income—whatever they earn on an average day of work, nothing more (well, if they insist . . .) and nothing less. What we can't raise that way, we'll earn through other means. And we will keep trying to obtain grants from foundations, even though our commitment to no fees, no third-party reimbursement, and no malpractice insurance will probably continue to inhibit traditional funding sources.

Once we open, we estimate an annual operating budget of $1 to $1.5 million, depending on donations. This wide variance will cover unknowns. We would like to give each staff person $3,000 a year beyond room and board, or $120,000 for the total staff. We estimate our annual food budget at $300,000 to $350,000 a year. The remaining costs will be for medications, medical supplies, farming needs, subscriptions to professional periodicals, household supplies, telephone, and electricity. Incidentals probably will cost more than $200,000 a year. After the buildings are finished, we will need a large amount of furniture and equipment, much of which will be donated. We will continue to apply for grants for specific items, since foundations often prefer to give money for equipment rather than for bricks and mortar. We cannot project exactly what our expenses will be; we must test the water. But we are confident that we can operate for less than $1.5 million a year.

We will "earn" this sum by donations primarily from our mailing list—now 6,500 names, with 10,000 names as a short-term goal. We also will sell our arts and crafts as well as commissioned pieces by artists who have promised to make pieces for us each year. If these sources fall short, we will seek outside work to subsidize Gesundheit, as we have done in the past. Our land is held as a land trust, and all incoming funds, from outside jobs and from donations, go to Gesundheit Institute, which is organized as a tax-free charitable entity. Our ultimate fantasy is to have a trust fund that will provide for all of Gesundheit's annual needs.

We intend to provide a very high quality of care at a small cost compared with other facilities. Considering what we have accomplished to date, there is every reason to believe we can do so. The bottom line is that this is not one man's story or creation but a total group effort toward peace. We have opened our lives and hearts to thousands of people, and the feedback has been overwhelmingly positive. We have received enormous encouragement to continue our efforts to help the world become a healthier, more loving place.

The Architect's Vision

Recently, Dave Sellers, the architect for the Gesundheit Institute, led a design charette—a weeklong brainstorming and creation session—for the hospital. Following is Dave's vision of the project.

One evening, a good many months after the design of the Gesundheit hospital had begun, my gaze settled on an aerial photograph of the Gesundheit land. In the picture, the sun cast long shadows that separated the limestone hills and ravines from the large meadow at their base, creating distinct forms. As I looked at them, these abstract shapes suddenly merged into a huge land-fish—and this fish was smiling the widest grin I'd ever seen. Right there in front of me was this one-thousand-foot-long fish made of trees, rocks, and hillside that had been eroded tens of thousands of years ago by glacial decline and earthly wild beginnings. In that moment I saw that the hospital would stand right at the opening of this fish's smiling mouth, the buildings rolling across the landscape like the sound of laughter.

The first time I ever heard of Gesundheit or even spoke to Patch was when—out of the blue—he called my office in Vermont to congratulate me on having been selected as the architect for the hospital. In the next breath, he informed me that I needed to get to the building site in West Virginia, meet everyone, and begin work as soon as possible. This first conversation consisted of bellowing laughter and specific project details. Patch explained that he wanted a hospital to be built with chandeliers strong enough to swing on, with trap doors in the library, and with slides from every level. He wanted a movie theater, stages, costume rooms, and gardens—lots of gardens. His main message to me then—and now—was that the hospital should be the best thing I had ever done. "Make it silly," he said, "and don't worry about anything, you will get all the support you need."

Gesundheit was originally conceived as an all-encompassing hospital that would offer free health care with a smile. Over the years the concept has evolved into Gesundheit being an institute for healing and for living life fully—having symptoms are simply a ticket to this university of life. The Institute will offer free outpatient care to the regional community. Gesundheit will also offer specialized clinics for Alzheimer's patients and for ear, eyes, nose, and throat imbalances. In addition, the Institute will have rooms and other spaces for meditating, dancing, and play, a theater, a center for social change, a library, and a school for children of patients, staff, and some members of the community-at-large. Gesundheit will welcome resident artists and thinkers to stay and share their gifts. They, in turn, will be nurtured

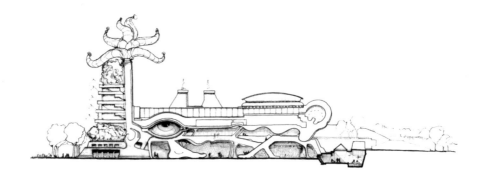

COURTYARD ELEVATION OF GESUNDHEIT HOSPITAL
(ILLUSTRATION BY DAVID SELLERS)

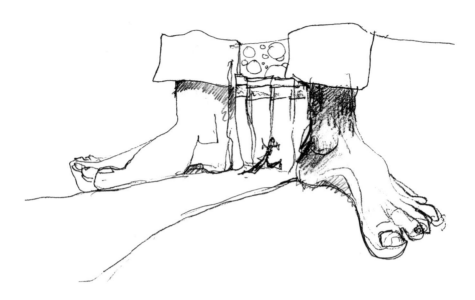

Clinic entrance

(Illustration by David Sellers)

and cared for by the Gesundheit staff. The structures are designed to help people connect to larger life processes and to better understand the functioning of the bodily organs that they have come to heal.

To reflect the evolving scope of the project, the Institute is now envisioned as a community of buildings. Instead of one hospital standing alone in a meadow, Gesundheit is now designed as two rows of buildings—a kind of village—gathered around a shared courtyard, and connected by an underground tunnel. On the courtyard side of the buildings, earth is mounded up to the roof level. From the main entrance the buildings appear as a series of roof shapes stepping up and down with only the Outpatient Center doors extending out through a gap in the earthen mounds.

Gesundheit will have two distinct but interdependent facilities. On the east side of the courtyard, running north to south, will be a series of buildings making up the Outpatient Center. New arrivals will enter the Center between a pair of huge feet at a break in the earth mounds. They will enter into a three-story light-filled domed room. This central hub will connect to all the outpatient clinics. Each of the eight examining rooms will have a special West Virginian theme, familiar to the patient and designed to help ease them into the Gesundheit

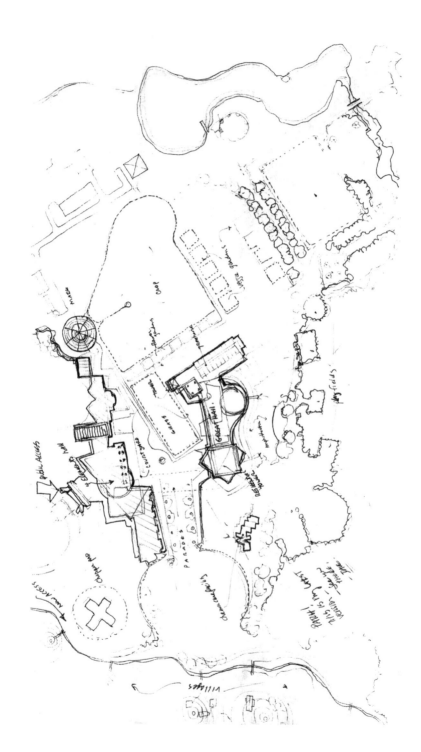

SITE PLAN FOR GESUNDHEIT HOSPITAL

(ILLUSTRATION BY DAVID SELLERS)

world. The Outpatient Center will be a fully-equipped regional facility, capable of handling all aspects of rural medicine on a drop-in or scheduled-appointment basis. Services will include emergency care, minor surgery, x-ray, ophthalmology, gynecology, dentistry, acupuncture, and allergy care. There will be beds for patients and for half of the staff, as well as special healing rooms, fun rooms (unusual spaces easily convertible to different experiences), and rooms dedicated to the four elements of life: fire, water, air, and earth.

At the southern end of the Outpatient Center will be a building standing alone—a chapel for birthing and dying. This is currently conceived as a large glass, greenhouse-like building. There will be a birthing tank at ground level. Overhead will be a large glass dome. People can raise themselves up and have whatever they imagine— such as their dying wish—projected on the dome surrounding them. A path will extend westward from this building, moving into a large field of wheat. Travelers will be led gradually lower until they are at eye-level with the plants.

On the opposite side of the Outpatient Center will be a series of buildings that celebrate such daily processes as harvesting, eating, and digesting, as well as providing services for chronic sensory imbalances. As in the Outpatient Center, these buildings will have earth mounded along most of the noncourtyard side. The structure of the main spaces will be similar to the bones in a bird's wing. Each strut and beam will serve a distinct purpose as they zing around, holding up stairs, slides, skylights, and clinics.

At the southernmost end will be a tower of showers, as well as the rest of the bedrooms for staff and patients. The top of the tower will be a combination water storage tank and lookout. Plants native to the area will grow around the water tower and trellis, keeping the water cool. On the very top, a box of inflatable shapes will be stored for a "jack-in-the-box" type of display for special events. These will inflate to give the tower top a goofy foolscap. Below and alongside the tower will be a large greenhouse where tanks overflowing with plants will convert the gray water and raw sewage into fresh water and a nutrient-rich compost that in turn will be spread over the gardens to become food again. The shape of the greenhouse will resemble a sphinx crouching at the base of the tower. The interior will resemble the cavernous interior of Monstro (the whale inside of whom Pinocchio was trapped). This is meant to visually and experientially connect the function of the room with a memory-shape

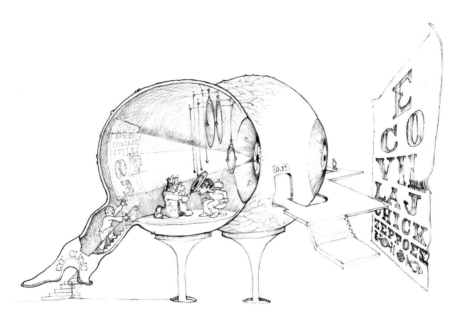

INTERIOR OF EYE EXAMINATION ROOM
(ILLUSTRATION BY JOHN CONNELL)

related to it. North of the greenhouse and tower will be the kitchens. Here staff and patients alike will prepare food harvested from the Gesundheit gardens. Alongside the kitchens will be a basilica-shaped dining hall, structured with forty-foot trees—branches and bark intact—that will be harvested from the adjacent forest. Areas where the branches connect will create bridges and lookouts, lofts and balconies. There will be an enormous fireplace at one end of the building and a floor above for dancing and other recreation.

North of the dining hall will be the Ear, Eye, Nose, and Throat Clinic. Each of these examining rooms will be designed to help visitors understand how the organs that they have come to heal actually function. For example, in the ear examination room they will brush up against a tympanic membrane (or ear drum) the size of an actual kettle drum. When they need medical attention for their eyes, they will enter a room shaped like an enormous eyeball. They'll also be able to reach out and touch the massive elements that transfer light to electrical impulses.

The space between the two rows of buildings will create a series of distinct courtyards. The first of these will be a circle defined by

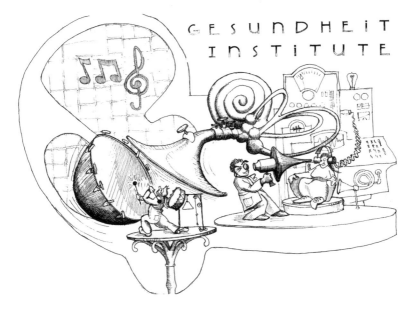

INTERIOR OF EAR EXAMINATION ROOM
(ILLUSTRATION BY JOHN CONNELL)

mounds of earth that taper from the north end of the buildings to the ground. A wedge-shaped courtyard will proceed from the perimeter of the circle through the two rows of buildings and to the entrance of the Outpatient Center. Here the wedge will flare open and step down into a square, gravel courtyard. (Underneath these steps, a tunnel will connect the Outpatient Center to the rest of the Institute.) Within the larger gravel courtyard will be a long, perfectly flat rectangle of grass, the site for daily fun and games.

The space between the buildings and the hills will form another series of outdoor rooms. Between the dining hall and the hill will be an amphitheater with terraced earth for seats and the hills as a backdrop for the stage. Between the kitchen and the hills will be the herb gardens. Carved out of the tree line will be several circular and rectangular playing fields.

Other landscape forms will include the existing man-made lake to the south and gardens between the lake and the greenhouse. Between these gardens and the hills will be a series of larger fields surrounded by trees. The last of these will be a large, square field surrounded by a gravel walkway. A path will wander through the lower portions of the hills, connecting remote waterfalls, special trees, and wildflower glades. The upper hills are off-limits to humans in respect for the privacy of other species living there.

As seen from the air, the overall site appears as a giant laughing clown, rolling out of the mouth of the laughing fish. The round Birthing-and-Dying Chapel is the eye, the large field beside it the nose, and the gardens below the nose a giant mustache and smile.

The rapidly emerging consciousness of ecological balance, regional responsibility, community values, the reemergence of the appreciation of craftsmanship, and above all the fostering of individual responsibility and freedoms in a garden of laughter are all ingredients in the soup of

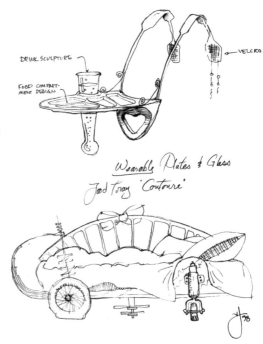

HOSPITAL EQUIPMENT

(ILLUSTRATION BY JOHN CONNELL)

the Gesundheit Institute. The first phase of construction will be to build the Outpatient Center and the living, cooking, and dining facilities. Building these structures will help us to know how to best approach the second phase. As it grows, Gesundheit will self-correct and forge new connections. The process of sifting through all these variables will bring on spurts of unannounced clarity and inspiration. To me the design process is like watching a deer run through grass that reaches over its head. Now and then it leaps high into the air, looking around for bearing, then drops back down to dash through the maze of grass before it leaps once again, realigning itself, repeating this process until the meadow is finally crossed.

11 • Living on the Land

Kathy Blomquist

Wandering, wandering, wanting it all . . .
a curious soul astray.
I ran with a passionate story.
I ran for the wisdom and glory.
As a child my dreams ran wild . . .
                                        k. d. lang and Ben Mink

Dream. Dream wild. Extremely wild dreams. Somewhere back there is a wild seed waiting. Of that I am sure.

Dream. Dream wild. Extremely wild dreams. Somewhere back there is a wild seed waiting. Of that, I am sure. Go and take a look. Take another look and bring your keenest sense. Sniff what you see. Hear what you feel. Grab a rake and a pail of water and ponder some. Pick up that wild seed and find a very, very convenient place to plant it, for throughout your days here you will need to keep it much closer than you are used to. Do not worry about what it will become or how you will coax it there. Truly, it will grow from this moment on. It's up to you.

Well-beings depend on these seeds. For all the attention you will now give this seed, it will tend you three hundred times

171

over with plenty remaining to take care of the other pioneers, probing their forgotten seeds. It's up to you.

Psssst . . . you are not alone.

Come run wild with other idealists and put a few of your ideals to work. Pick up the phone and give us a call.

Since 1980, thousands of pioneering people have called to volunteer their time and skills on the land site where the hospital of Patch's wild dream-seed has been planted amidst an eclectic community cluster. Volunteers come from all over the world for a range of reasons, with hearts full of goodwill and service.

Gesundheit Institute, a project unleashed by Patch Adams in medical school, is an experience in holism based on the belief that one cannot separate the health of the individual from the health of the family, the community, and the world. In 1980 Gesundheit purchased 310 acres from a lumber company in Pocahontas County, near Hillsboro, West Virginia. Located in the heart of the Appalachian Mountains, surrounded by national and state forests, and at the headwaters of eight rivers, the land inspires a natural and diverse brand of creativity and stewardship. The hills are some of the oldest in the world, home to caves and caverns and a wide range of flora and fauna. The down payment for the land was provided by a core of eight wild dreamers and the property came with a small farmhouse, a large barn, and several outbuildings.

Activity on the land was limited from 1980–1983, but in 1983 there was a jump in funds and activity which prompted the start of construction on our first new building—a 6,500 square-foot workshop. Since then a multitude of projects have been completed in a grassroots fashion to enhance the property and its people. Two wells were dug in 1988. Before that time a fickle spring delivered water by a gravity-fed system which meant that sometimes there was running water—and sometimes there was not. Imagine having to haul all the cooking, drinking, cleaning, and bathing water for a group of twenty hardworking volunteers in mid-July! Imagine how frequently the exposed, black piping froze up in the winter! And it wasn't until 1990 that plumbing brought the first flush-toilets as a waste management option. Early land-dwellers were certainly pioneers of spirit and vision, holding passionately onto the wildest dream—the dream of building a free hospital on 310 acres of rural land in rustic conditions, with primitive facilities, and with no money. Where do you begin? And how do you sustain? At Gesundheit, village pioneers began with humble homesteading, working side by side with volunteers to build, remodel, garden, cook, clean, and misbehave. These pioneers sustained themselves with their belief in the joy of service for a higher purpose and through collective effort. In that spirit we have continued.

Our main on-site work in West Virginia has been to look after what we have, to restore what we can, and finally to introduce new elements into well-functioning systems. To date, Gesundheit has completed a three-story workshop building with a basement and fully equipped woodworking studio, a three-acre lake, a two-mile woodland trail, a greenhouse and porch additions to the farmhouse, toolsheds, a three-season dwelling for long-term volunteers, decking platforms for our yurts, and preliminary landscaping and intensive organic gardening.

Our main focus, along with building and maintaining our community's physical foundations, has been delving further into the ongoing development of our human design—that being how we all interact when we come together to work and play and live. The purpose of our volunteer program is to contribute to the mental, spiritual, and physical foundation of the Gesundheit Institute, and to participate in building a larger community committed to making a difference. People came to Gesundheit because they believe in our *vision* to build a free hospital where all healing arts are welcome and all healers, including the patients, serve together in a rural community setting. Our hope is that they go home with this *mission*: to inspire others to change their world through relentless, joyful, sustaining service. There are three key ways we do this:

- **Working with the land**—the physical tasks of maintaining and consciously designing the natural and built environments.

- **Working with ourselves**—the individual's tasks of sustaining a dynamic level of fitness—body, mind, heart, and soul.

- **Working with each other**—the group's task of creating a collective consciousness amidst unity and diversity.

Gesundheit attracts a blessed mix of people who want to give, purely and truly. In order to host most effectively, we offer two volunteer options. The majority of people come for 1–2 weeks during our peak season, which runs from April to September. There is no selection process for the short-term volunteer, which means no one has to have any particular skills or abilities. We also host long-term volunteers up to six months at a time. Most of these volunteers have been with us previously for a two-week visit, have a specific skill necessary to the functioning of our community, and are available to dive deep into our experiment. We spend more time with this group, working out details and expectations to ensure the best fit for every-one. Staff positions might also be considered volunteer positions, although we get monthly stipends based on our personal financial needs. Stipends cover the most basic personal needs while the com-munity provides all other essentials—food, shelter, and fun. New staff members actually experience one full year as a staff apprentice before being considered full-time. Due to space and money and year-round need, these positions have been very limited.

The land has operated like a summer camp for alternative seekers and idealists who are eager for fun. On any given day during our season, four to forty people live, work, and play together. Volunteers work according to our needs, as well as to their skills and interests. All meals and communal lodging are provided without charge. Each spring we raise two yurts—round Mongolian style tents—and set them on top of wooden platforms next to an outhouse and solar shower. We live simply and remotely in the country with hot and cold running water, electricity, and telephones.

The organized work week runs Monday through Friday, with weekends free for volunteers to explore the area. New volunteers arrive on weekends by train, plane, or automobile, and each Sunday evening we gather all volunteers and staff to make a round of intro-ductions and present projects for the week. It's a chance for our project leaders to give a rousing pitch for their work/play (plork) activity—one that will set fresh recruits slurping with plork delight. An orientation Monday morning goes over the nitty-gritties of how we will actually move and groove with each other.

Our days begin at seven A.M. with a mighty wake-up call from the conch shell. After breakfast, volunteers sign up for the plork activity of their choice and then everyone plugs in. We all participate in kitchen work, as well as in a general clean-up on Friday afternoon. Many people consider the kitchen to be the "Center of the Universe."

Indeed, a large bulk of our time is spent in this area which also serves as a place for a lively exchange of information, opinions, and music. All our land-dwellers help run the kitchen, signing up on Sunday night for the following week's meals. We do our best to accommodate everyone's dietary preferences, allergies, and levels of ability in cooking for a large group.

Evening activities are a gift of spontaneity and improvisation. Some folks offer bodywork or drumming; others lead workshops or make a sweat lodge. Maybe you'd like to hike our mountain trail or swing in the hammocks.

Use of drugs—specifically nonprescription, illegal drugs—is prohibited. If you are or have been chemically dependent in any way, we ask you not to consume at Gesundheit. Volunteers who abuse themselves or others will be asked to leave.

Don't leave your kids home alone. We love kids and can usually integrate their care into the flow of our program. But please do leave your pets at home.

So what does this all mean? We take our play as seriously as our work and keep our work as ridiculous as our play. And we actually get things done! So prepare yourself for a plork-style that's a little crazy, and a little zany.

We hold everyone responsible for their own delight. In other words, you create your own experiences here. We strongly encourage people to be themselves and to ASK when questions or concerns pop up. Communication is the most important ingredient in our Gesundheit soup.

In this context, a lot of healing and powerful moments can happen. We allow for such expression and renewal. At the same time, this project is not one that offers sanctuary or retreat as a primary focus, since expectations for being able to handle what can be demanding work or community process are part of the program. Therefore, if people are in crisis or need a lot of nurturing, our volunteer program probably would not be appropriate. We stimulate dialogue, expose people to new ideas, listen intently to each other's delights, drink up each task, speak out and go directly to the source of conflict, exchange a few secrets, hug and sing and ponder, find our fun, and above all be who we are and encourage that trueness in others.

As you might expect, being a staff-resident on the land in West Virginia has been an extraordinary adventure. I believe I was given, by nature and by nurture, a firm foundation from which to explore this kind of life work. I grew up in Hallock, Minnesota, a predominantly Scandinavian town of one thousand in the northwestern nook of the state. My notions of genuine community are rooted in this rural midwestern culture. Through family and friends, from baptism to graduation, I formulated a belief system about myself and the world that only lately have I fully realized and honored. Seeded in my Scandinavian heritage is an array of virtuous verbs to live by—trust, believe, work, dedicate, help, cooperate. I didn't grow up feeling victimized by society. In fact, in that small town with a community of caring people surrounding me, I grew up feeling fundamentally curious about society's design. Motivation to act has become influenced by what is right with our present design, not by what is wrong.

With the self-reliance of a good Norwegian, I've spent most of my life work pursuing matters of the heart and searching for genuine insights into how people work, grow, and care for each other. I became a registered nurse, creating a third generation of nurses in our family. Since then, my unfolding odyssey has been ever more expansive as a result of the strong bond I have with my first family and community which by example taught me to be kind, caring, friendly, reliant, and respectful. Thanks Mom and Dad.

When you have at your side virtuous verbs to live by, there comes a time when the animated adjectives collected along the way demand declaration. I moved to West Virginia in 1993 to help manage the volunteer program at Gesundheit and little did I know . . . I knew so little about what I had leapt into. Now, I know why I leapt. My wild, wandering curious soul wanted to run. And a forgotten seed wanted some attention. So with tenacious belief in the essentially good, kind, and compassionate, I discovered I could express myself even further. It was time to actively infuse robust trust, passionate work, voracious help, delirious dedication, and perpetual belief. Uff Da. (Ask a Norwegian.)

I love journeys. I love quests. I love that it is my job to journey and quest with many others on passionate pursuits and mundane madness. Clearly, people want shifts in many areas of their lives, and within most aspects of their communities. Promoting these dialogues with our volunteers becomes an every minute experience—wherever we may be. We may begin a conversation about problems in health care delivery while in the kitchen chopping onions. By the time our soup is ready, we've moved from a general conversation to a more specific unfolding of one another's personal beliefs and values. In fact, in these dialogues wild dream-seeds can be uncovered and playfulness unzipped. This is the real joy of the journey we're on with all the people we host and live with—the journey to alien worlds of play until the playlien in you wakes up.

Amidst the growing number of movements serving community, the Global Ecovillage Network (GEN) of projects has emerged as a small group of representatives from ecovillage projects around the world that work together to promote and explore low-impact, sustainable-community design. Gesundheit has plunged into the EEK-O part of this village movement. Based on the principle that the health of the individual cannot be separated from the health of the rest of our EEKosystem, we at Gesundheit aim to engage ourselves as a holistic medical community with the Global Ecovillage Network in order to provide a forum for sharing knowledge and integrating principles of sustainability—ecological, spiritual, economical, and social. In an ecovillage, human activities are integrated with the natural world in such a way that human development may be sustained indefinitely. And in an EEKovillage, human beings will integrate with their ridiculous natural selves in such a way that joy and service will be sustained most definitely.

To my knowledge, no fully functioning ecovillages exist on the planet. In other words, we are at the conception of definition and declaration for the modern era, which is a very exciting position to be in. *Ecovillages and Sustainable Communities* outlines six main challenges facing visionaries as they work to merge ideals with practical matters:*

> 1. *The biosystem*: How will we preserve natural habitats on the land?
> 2. *The built environment*: What design principles will emerge, utilizing ecologically friendly materials?
> 3. *The economic system*: Are there useful alternatives to the money system?
> 4. *The governance*: How will decisions be made, conflicts resolved?
> 5. *The glue—shared values and vision*: What is the appropriate balance of unity and diversity?
> 6. *The whole system*: How will a right relationship to all systems be maintained in order to develop at a sustainable pace?

* Ecovillage and Sustainable Communities. (Findham, Scotland: Findhorn Press, 1996).

Knowing what is wrong with these systems is easy. The hard part is knowing what else to do. Permaculture principles provide a practical way to unfold an ecovillage using a design system that meets basic human needs while preserving natural ecosystems. It is applicable to food, water, shelter, energy, social, and economic systems. Permaculture is a "way of organizing knowledge, a connecting system that integrates science, art, politics, anthropology, sociology, psychology, and the diverse experiences and resources available in any community."*

Challenges abound and overlap as we begin to contemplate how our particular core members will implement sustainable practices. How will we steward our land? What sort of appropriate technology will we use in our structures? How will we handle our money and make sound financial decisions? Who will make decisions? Who will make peace? How will we practice diversity and share unity? Will we model these complexities with the simplicity necessary to stimulate change that can be sustained? Did we just bewitch all of the above with fun and delight? Did we promise to forgive ourselves and others for the first, second, or three-hundredth mistake? Designing our village cluster has become an invigorating artistic attempt to sculpt an improved society. This creativity spawns joyful service and will chaperone us through the next unfolding phases.

Our volunteers keep reminding me how differently rich we can be and still behold what is good and most kind. And although they haven't found the strawbale walls of a hospital yet, they are given the type of hospitality that has almost been forgotten. Be bombastically nice, make intimate friends, welcome a motley stranger, and run with playlien fun. These are the wildest ideals.

I love this journey.

I love this quest.

Now go on, get to it, pick a vivacious verb to live by and plant it next to your wildly seeded dream. It's up to you.

Here's to all idealists and momentarians: Come Volunteer! Call or write *at least* one month in advance. Vavoom!

Gesundheit Institute
HC 64 Box 167
Hillsboro, WV 24946
(304) 653-4338

*(*Living Community: A Permaculture Case Study at Sol y Sombre.* Ben Haggard)

12 · Light a Candle: How Can I Help?

Medicine practiced as a business hurts everyone. The true rewards of medicine come from helping others and from self-discovery. . . . Service is essential to healing and the pathway to inner peace.

While Gesundheit Institute is not the single answer to America's health care needs, we hope it will stimulate people involved in health care—or any endeavor—to join with their cohorts and ask "What do we want? What are our dreams and fantasies? How do we band together and work with our communities to make them a reality?" Do not be daunted by the enormity of the problems associated with health care delivery or with the lethargic pace of change. If you find people of like mind and desire and are willing to devote your life to a goal, all your dreams—about a new health care system or a new society—are possible. Anticipate a million mistakes and disappointments, but feel the thrill of the quest—belief in the possibility is itself invigorating. The key for the long haul is realizing that tiny steps, taken a day at a time, will erode gargantuan problems. The simplest, cheapest affirmative step you can take right away is to first clean your own house. Discard any negative attitudes and feeling of limitations that have held you back from taking action. Begin to appreciate the miracle of life; enjoy the world's many treasures and be thankful for them. Focus on your sense of belonging to all humanity and, indeed, to all forms of life.

What Health Care Professionals Can Do

I have some suggestions for health care professionals that are based on many years of experience and observation. Ultimately I hope you will come up with your own approaches to issues relevant to your communities and practices. To improve the general climate of medical care and to move medicine out of the business sector, spend some time thinking about health care needs and discussing them with colleagues who are involved in all phases of care. Reflect on the dialogue and start to build a foundation for the changes you all believe are important.

Be open to all healing arts. Spend one day a month with someone you've heard about who represents a different healing tradition, and try to establish a sense of peership among these other healers.

Become involved with your community. As you work to convert medicine from a business to a community service, encourage legislation, such as that passed by Virginia and other states, that exempts free medical service from malpractice suits. Be patient; this process may take many years.

Establish networks of volunteers to help people find work, shelter, friends, and whatever else they need. The true resources of even a poor community are grossly underused. Interdependence and helping seem natural in times of disaster, like an earthquake or a flood. We must recognize that a more subtle disaster is upon us now and muster our resources accordingly.

Health care professionals can also take steps to move medicine from a hierarchy of power and prestige to one of a friendly team spirit. Encourage staff at all levels to socialize more. Downplay the use of titles. Eat with all the people you work with, whether out at a restaurant or in each others' homes. Be friendly at work; for example, in the nursing station, find an appropriate demeanor that allows hugging and massaging to occur on a regular basis. Find like-minded colleagues who are willing to serve on "hug patrol" for both staff and patients.

To lighten up what has traditionally been a somber environment, try to create an office, clinic, or hospital that is fun to work in and to visit as a patient. Be enthusiastic and friendly toward all people. Integrate art and humor into the context of the facility. Set aside places—dining and even play areas—for staff and patients to get together socially. Find alternatives to those awful hospital gowns.

Physicians and nurses, as a part of or along with your regular jobs, you can spend one or two afternoons a week making house calls. Visit several patients or—even better—spend the entire time with one patient or family in their home. Share a meal with them. Devote at least one day a week to free care in your clinic or other clinics. Above all, as you become a voice for necessary social change within your profession or outside it, enlist patients and citizens in your actions and dialogues for a better health care system.

Hospital administrators can also work to bring about change by setting an example for diminished hierarchy and bureaucracy in the health care system. Initiate open forums for all staff and your community. Work with legislatures and medical societies on long-term planning of a service-oriented model for health care. In the meantime, devote some thought and energy to making your hospital a more hospitable place, and help midwife your hospital's transition. Set aside space for an experimental "goofy" ward where staff and patients can enjoy humor and fun. Enlist community artists to help create a more beautiful, uplifting environment in your facility.

A Message for Concerned Medical Students

Medical education can be a stressful experience. Some students find the academics gargantuan; others are overwhelmed by the costs. But the most disconcerting feedback I have heard is students' depression and anxiety about the climate in which health care is practiced in today's society. They are finding that a joyous, service-oriented practice in hospitals is rare. Economics and management often appear to come before patient care, and competition seems to have replaced cooperation among many health care professionals.

These suggestions are for the medical student who yearns for a thrilling, heartfelt medical education, who is pursuing his or her studies in joyous anticipation of a lifetime of service to humankind. Always remember to assert your own motivations, respect your wisdom, and be confident that *you* can make your life an exuberant adventure.

Never become complacent about the miracle of life. As you explore the glorious mechanisms of the body, let the understanding of their processes electrify you with wonder and curiosity. Live in awe and let *that* be the focus of your education, *not* your grades, which tell you nothing about the kind of doctor you will be. When I was in medical school, I told my professors never to notify me about my grades unless I failed. This became very freeing.

Don't wait until you are on the wards to develop and practice your interviewing skills. Start now! Interview everybody in as much depth as you dare. Medicine's fundamental thrill is intimacy. To achieve it, you must practice interviewing a wide variety of people. Try calling wrong numbers, talking to friends, talking to everyone. Find the kind of demeanor that delights others so much that they tell you their stories. Be ecstatic when people give you their trust, love, and intimacy. Let this journey with others fill you with the excitement of finding new friends.

Become involved in the politics of medicine from the beginning. Join the American Holistic Medical Association (AHMA), American Medical Student Association (AMSA), Office of Student Representatives of the Association of American Medical Colleges (OSR), American Medical Association (AMA), American Academy of Family Physicians (AAFP), and similar organizations. Attend meetings, especially the big ones, and talk to everybody. Many of your colleagues are thinking about the same issues you are. You may find support that will help your ideal medical practice germinate and thrive.

Cultivate relationships with health care professionals and professors you respect. Establish a lively dialogue. Invite yourself to their homes. Ask to come into their practices. Cultivate the same intimacy with aides, orderlies, and nurses as with physicians and patients. Wherever you go in life, friendliness will make your days exciting.

Build support groups for study and play. Find kindred souls and fantasize about your medical interests and futures. Practice being deep and intimate with one another; hold nothing back. If you can, share ideas with other groups. From these contacts can come medical partners for life, wherever you settle.

Focus on medicine as service. Medicine practiced as a business hurts everyone. The true rewards of medicine come from helping others and from self-discovery. Giving is intoxicating; it produces intimacy as a byproduct. Brace yourself for an avalanche of love.

Do not let the cost of education paralyze you. Enjoy the privilege of being in school; when you finish, you will pay your loans back as soon as you can. If you choose service-oriented medicine, its gift will be payback enough until funds come in. Don't let debt trap you in a repugnant practice; there is no debtor's prison anymore. Let creativity and exploration help you. Community support can be a key.

Cultivate outside interests. You are not merely a doctor—you are a person who has studied medicine! Nurture all of your loves and experiment with ways of integrating them with your medicine. Weave these interests into the relationships you have with your patients and be open to learning from them. You will thrive on the bonds that form.

Do not sacrifice your family for your medical career. What you learn from keeping your family life vibrant will help you serve your patients. Plan time out from work and study to spend with your family. Cherish your mate, lovers, children, and parents, and feel the great health their love gives you. Make your friends part of your family, too.

Above all, fantasize your most outlandish medical dreams. Your degree in medicine is a license to choose exactly how you want to practice. The only limiting factors will be your fears and lack of imagination. Flock together and soar! And as you grow and learn, please share your feedback, suggestions, and dialogue with us and with your contemporaries so that together we can create a medical celebration.

What About the Rest of Us?

How can people outside the medical profession light the way toward a better health care system? The most important steps begin with yourself. Learn to like yourself, for you are your own most constant companion. Try to experience life as a journey toward your fondest dreams. This is the surest path to personal happiness, which, I believe, is the foundation of good health.

One of the best ways to develop self-esteem is to cultivate friendships. Your love of yourself and of your most intimate friends will grow as you tell one another how wonderful you are. Learn how to play; having fun develops self-esteem as you bring joy to yourself and to others, making more friends in the process. Try playing in the mud or wearing your underwear on the outside of your clothes. Rent funny movies. Smell more roses. Sing aloud in public.

Try new ways of living. Take a month off work each year, if you can. Start growing some of the food you eat, whether in a window box or in a garden plot you cultivate lovingly with your own hands. Celebrate and diversify your hobbies; they are great sources of joy and self-esteem. One small but revolutionary lifestyle change is to turn off the television set. Try to reduce your viewing hours by half and use that time to read or play with your kids. When you do watch television, tune in to public television programs or exercise while you watch. The object is not to eliminate television watching entirely but to reduce the number of hours spent in passivity.

Take better care of yourself: eat nutritious foods, walk more, and exercise your mind along with your body. Spend more time enjoying nature and the arts, and give vent to your curiosity, imagination, and creativity. Positive changes in personal health behavior are the best way to achieve genuine health care reform. Such changes could help create a world in which physicians and other health care professionals are no longer primarily mechanics fixing breakdowns, but gardeners nurturing growth.

Balance your personal life with your work life by taking more time for family and loved ones—they are the antidotes to loneliness and the key to a happy life. Find small ways to bring joy to others: be friendly while waiting in line at the supermarket, smile at strangers, play with children, learn to give massages. Learn to enjoy the company of both men and women, as well as people whose lifestyles are vastly different from yours. Welcome cultural diversity and explore people of other races, colors, and creeds. Talk about and celebrate your differences. Study geography to learn about the world and its people and to promote environmental and global connectedness.

Service is essential to healing and the pathway to inner peace. Take an interest in health care in your community and volunteer your time and skills to hospitals, clinics, nursing homes, hospices, and other caregiving organizations. Seek cooperative arrangements by inviting new people to visit your home and share activities or to live with you in single-parenting or co-housing situations. Your efforts will help create a stronger community as well as a healthier health care system.

Become involved in the political process at the local, community, and state levels. Learn about environmental and other issues vital to a healthy society and world. Vote, write letters to policy makers and legislators, and join special interest groups. Rather than trying to find a way to finance the existing health care system, those of you who are legislators can support new service-oriented models based on creative visions for an ideal health care system, especially those that emphasize wellness and prevention. Work to create a system based not on powerful interest groups but on what is truly needed; reduce the influence wielded over your decisions by insurance and pharmaceutical companies.

Social revolutionaries have always come up with scores of suggestions for how to change the world. Make your own list; having made it, let your voice be heard. Invent your own ways to take action and you will prevent passivity and its devastating offspring—boredom, fear, and loneliness—from taking over your life. Experience life as a wondrous, zestful journey. Dare to dream—as we at Gesundheit have dreamed—of better health for individuals, families, communities, and the world. Your dreams will keep hope, and the possiblity of change, alive.

13 · Passion and Persistence

I don't want people to be amazed by our passion and persistence, but inspired by us to work long and hard for what they believe in.

Passion and persistence can change the world! I'm talking about hanging in there *joyfully*—that last word is extremely important.

I'm traveling around quite a lot these days, both to generate enthusiasm for building our hospital and to stimulate living a life of service. And whether I'm speaking to hospital CEOs or to university students, my audience is often left in a state of amazement—amazement caused not by our ideals or the breadth of our work, but by the passion and persistence we display in pursuing our goals and in living our lives. And this disturbs me. I don't want people to be amazed at our passion and persistence, but inspired by us to work long and hard for what they believe in. I have a tremendous desire for social change and see passion and persistence as the key to creating change.

Our society, bereft of self-esteem, is being suffocated by its own sense of powerlessness. What I want to do is to make passion and persistence so common-

186

place that they no longer are even interesting or strange, because they have become the rule rather than the exception. These qualities should not be seen as attributes of special people who are blessed enough to possess them, but rather as extremely important tools for change.

To show you the excellent company that such traits as passion and persistence keep, I need only to list a few of their equally well-known cousins: intensity, inspiration, obsession, commitment, insanity, craziness, relentlessness, dauntlessness, rage, energy, and concern.

I'm not sure passion and persistence can be taught. In our community I used to try. I'd collect all kinds of jigsaw puzzles—the harder the better. I would say to people, "You want to learn passion and persistence? Then do this puzzle and don't get up until it is done. Don't even *want* to get up until it is done." Passion and persistence can be inspired, studied, desired, pursued. I think that's why I am who I am. I consider myself a designed person—meaning I don't perform very many unintentional acts. I'm trying to be a person who might inspire passion. I get good feedback, which is why I do it. You can do the same thing for yourself. Get involved!

Can passion and persistence be found through revelation, vision, or rational thought? I think so. Shy and quiet people exhibit passion and persistence as deeply as the loud and obnoxious—though, to be sure, I'm more familiar with those falling into the latter category.

I believe passion and persistence are incompatible with, in fact dramatically damaged by, cynicism apathy, discouragement, and whining (cynicism and whining probably being my two biggest pet peeves). If you are going to be a social crusader, you must eliminate these things from your vocabulary and behavior. They are pernicious. They all kill the spirit of effort. When you use the language of these qualities, it results in an inertia so strong that it creates a strangling atmosphere of powerlessness.

Passion, of course, implies glorious scenes: the grandopening of the future Gesundheit facility, or getting a bill passed in Congress that you worked for ten years to push through. But this kind of passion needs no encouragement. The passion that tips the scale, the passion that makes the real difference, is the passion to endlessly hang posters—even one more time—or to call, yet again, another meeting where almost no one shows up, even though people promised to be there, and still find the ability to be feverishly enthusiastic for those two people who did show up. I'm talking about that passion that actually loves scutwork.

As a communitarian, you sometimes want to say, "What are the jobs that people see as the worst?" And then, after you've got your answers, find the seduction in those jobs that makes people love doing them. Now, that is passion!

I represent an extreme bias—mostly my own experience as a crazed person—but I think I can say without too much exaggeration that I have spent my entire fifty-plus years of life exploring passion and persistence, not only in myself, but in other people as well. Here are a few pointers on becoming a passionate and persistent individual:

• **Ground yourself in missions of higher good and service.** In my office at home, I have photos of murdered children and of children on the day they died of starvation. I have a personal ritual. I stand in front of these pictures until I am sobbing to remind myself that in my luxury, at this very second while I live in luxury, men are taking pleasure in torture. Ground yourself deeply in a mission for higher good.

• **Unite your mission with the miracle of life.** Unite your mission with your personal, perpetual experience of the miracle of life. Celebrate and be thankful that you have it together enough to step out of your selfish self, and have the opportunity to give yourself to others and to the world.

• **Make it fun!** As Emma Goldman said, "If I can't dance, I don't want to be part of your revolution!" Feel your path as a rich, varied, and uplifting experience. It needn't be my kind of fun— make it your own brand.

• **Persistence is a by-product of passion.** Wherever you see persistence, passion is at work. To me, passion feels like a surrender, a freedom from doubt, a zest for pursuit.

• **Live as close to your authentic self as you possibly can.** As a friend of mine says, "It's redundant to say 'authentic self' because self is authentic." Say what's on your mind—that day. No more lag time for perspective. Do what you want to do. No more sacrifice.

• **Find creativity in every act.** Don't ever sacrifice your need to be creative. Creativity is one of the greatest medicines ever. Exercise it in the way you wash dishes, in the way you walk down the street, and in the way you make art. Creativity is essential nourishment. It is not cute. It is not a luxury, as our government implies. It is the very soul of our sense of self-worth.

•**Responsibility, sacrifice, struggle, and whining hurt passion.**
These are horrible ways by which to motivate yourself. There's a
good chance that if you are motivated by a sense of responsibility,
sacrifice, and struggle, you will grow to blame or resent the very
thing you are passionate about. You'll start to see it as some kind of
excuse for what's not happening—or the reason for your pain
around it.

•**Passion is not a final product.** Passion is the name of a process.
This confusion in meaning is one reason why so many people quit
being passionate, or never even become part of a Big Dream.
People quit because they feel the process of achieving the final
product is too slow. Certainly the single most tragic occurrence in
Gesundheit's work has been the loss of great people because it's
taken so long to reach our final product. The statement "How is
Gesundheit doing?" always implies the final product of a finished
hospital, rather than the journey toward it. You must feel that
passion today, in the process—don't tie it to a finish line.

•**Invite cotravelers.** Cotravelers are the vital juice of any project.
Tell me this: Is there anything in your life more important than
your friends? Live your life that way! Commit yourself to your
friends and colleagues! They are your pillars of persistence.
Acknowledge them, support them, strive for the intimacy of your
wildest dreams with every human being you meet.

•**Live the life of an enthusiator.** A seducer. Yes, that is my job.
Pumping up and seducing. All of you should be working around
the clock, everyday for the rest of your life, fulfilling your dreams.
Not because you're paid to do it, but because you can't help it. It
feels that good.

•**Feel the thrill of the quest all the time.** Dream the impossible
dream, right the unrightable wrong. Yes, it's corny stuff, but also
the best.

•**See life itself as a break.** I'm not a break person. As Weird Al
Yankovich says, "I'll be mellow when I'm dead." I want you to
find so much delight with your cotravelers, so much thrill in the
quest, that a break is an irritation. Now if you need a break—and
this is Dr. Adams speaking—I want you to take one THAT DAY.
Don't put it off. I don't want you working under stress. In my

opinion, the reason there are so few social activists is that in the history of social activism, none of them ever look as if they are having any fun! It looks like only sacrifice and struggle. It looks like everyone you know who is doing it needs a break. Burnout? You know, we should be burned out from selfishness, from vacations, from breaks. Life—your life—needs to be designed so that the idea of a break is an unwelcome interruption. But until you reach that point, take a break on the day you need it.

• **Exercise your wonder, curiosity, and imagination at all times.**

• **Exercise as exercise.** Be physically fit. If you're not taking care of yourself, your community will have to take care of you. In order to be a passionate worker on a big project, you'd better stay physically fit, because accomplishing anything worthwhile is going to take a long time! Make fitness part of the ethic of your effort. Rest when you need it. Otherwise spend your time wisely.

• **Define success as something achievable.** For myself, I define success like this: Did I try? Did I give my time? Did I never give up? All of which are very easy to do. Do not put success in things or outcomes.

• **Don't borrow much money.** In the course of trying to build a free hospital, countless people have urged us to borrow money. The weight of borrowed money can cause you to lose your dream.

• **Delight in compromise wherever you can.** Have the shortest possible list of uncompromisable points. Say, "Sure. I like your way."

• **Be cautious about the power your passion brings.** Passionate people are given a lot of power in our society, whether they ask for it or not. Because we have so little self-esteem, such boredom and loneliness and fear, passion is extremely attractive. Be cautious.

At the age of eighty, the sculptor Henry Moore was asked what it was that he considered to be the secret to life. Moore's reply pretty much sums it up. "The secret of life is to have a task, something you devote your entire life to, something you bring everything to, every minute of the day for the rest of your life. And the most important thing is, it must be something you cannot possibly do."

Wheeeeeeeeeeeeeeeeeeeeee!

14 ⬩ Five Years Have Passed

Five years have passed, five summers,
with the length of five long winters . . .
William Wordsworth, "Tintern Abbey"

The book has really helped bring our ideas more clearly to a much wider audience all over the world. We get thousands of letters telling how our work has inspired similar projects and people—not just in the health field but in all human endeavors.

I wanted to write an addendum to catch up readers on what has been happening with Gesundheit these five years since the book was first printed. I wish I could say that the hospital has been built—or that at least it is going up as I write—but sadly, I cannot. What I can say is that many great things have happened for Gesundheit and we believe we are at a point where funding is imminent.

This hope comes largely because Universal Studios bought the movie rights to this book and in February 1998 they began shooting a film of my life with a December 1998 release-date scheduled. Robin Williams—much to my delight—will play me. All of us at Gesundheit have great hope that the movie will in some way promote joyful, relentless service. We also hope that the impact of a national movie can finally build our hospital.

191

Generous gifts, along with the making of the movie, led us in January 1998 to hold a design charrette (a major brainstorming session) for the hospital. This event felt like Gesundheit's finest hour. Led by our architect Dave Sellers, who has been involved in the project for sixteen years, over thirty of us met for a week in Warren, Vermont, working from early morning to late at night to design the first silly hospital. In attendance were ten of our staff (including four doctors and three nurses), another ten designers (including Jain Malkin, who has written the bible on hospital interior architecture; Doug Kelbaugh, Dean of the University of Michigan School of Architecture; Leslie Jacobs, hospital designer; John Connell, founder of Yestermorrow Design/Build School in Vermont; Daisy Rankin, an industrial designer from London; and many more brave creative minds), a performance art group, an environmentalist, and one of our big donors from Germany. At the end of the week I spoke before a packed house in the Warren Town Hall with a display of sixty drawings and models on hand for those in attendance to view.

Kathy Blomquist has been the manager at the building site these five years and she has brought great spark and progress to Gesundheit. She has spearheaded our commitment to being an example of environmental direction for sustainable human culture, and now we at Gesundheit insist upon our facility and community being what people in the environmental movement have termed an "ecovillage." Our decision to move in this direction was a crucial step for Gesundheit and has manifested in many ways—especially in our five years of exploration into permaculture. We also have twice hosted the Performers Workshop Ensemble's School for Designing Society and come to realize that the continued involvement of this school must be part of our final plans. We feel it is possible to teach people to be instruments for social change.

In these five years I have been much more active in lecturing and performing, and now have up to fifty possible presentations, having enhanced the scope and intelligence of the presentations through collaborating with a working partner, Susan Parenti, who for more than twenty years has been involved in social change through performance. We like to go to universities and lecture in classrooms all day and to the larger university community at night. If we're lucky we even go late into the night, talking with students on such vital subjects as friendship or how to follow your dreams. We have been asked to come to communities and help them move toward healthier ways of living together—and our work has expanded all over the world. Last year we brought our ideas to Poland, Sweden, Australia, New Zealand, Germany, Switzerland, Austria, Holland, England, Scotland, Canada, Russia, and Bosnia. Even medical students in Madagascar have told me how *Gesundheit!* has changed the way they look at medicine.

Our clowning work in Russia is now in its fourteenth year. This last year we took twenty-seven clowns ages 13–80 from five countries, thirteen of whom were repeat visitors. Five staff now lead these trips which have become so popular that we have added a spring trip. Our involvement with orphans brought to our attention the horrible abuses in Russian orphanages and for the last four years we have worked to build our own orphanage there. Our friend Maria from Moscow has worked so ardently for this, but we need support and hope people will help us make this orphanage a reality. Last year these trips brought twenty-two clowns to Bosnia. And every year we feel that our clowning work is expanding and influencing many spin-offs.

Gesundheit! has really helped bring our ideas more clearly to a much wider audience all over the world. We get thousands of letters telling how our work has inspired similar projects and people—not just in the health field but in all human endeavors. In the long run, providing this inspiration may be the most important consequence of our work. I suppose this inspiration is what has prompted the Peace Abbey to give us the Courage of Conscience Award and the Institute of Noetic Science's Temple Award for Creative Altruism.

These five years we have been very active in better developing the mechanics of our organization. We have devoted more effort to creating a participatory useful board of directors, as well as to establishing a much broader base of leadership. It is always important for a complex project that was begun by one person to work to eliminate that person's indispensability. These five years have brought the staff so close as friends and workers that my leadership no longer feels necessary for Gesundheit's survival. The people involved are why I stay with the project.

The saddest part of the story is that in June 1997, my wife Linda Edquist and I separated after twenty-six years. Linda and I started this work and her input over the years has been critical. I can never thank her enough. Linda, I salute the great gifts you've born for me and for Gesundheit. Neither of us would be what we are had you not been the giant that you are.

Bibliography:
A Booklover's Search for
Understanding and Ideas

Welcome to my library! Ever since my high school days, books and magazines have been to my mind what friends are in the flesh. Each and every one of these books and articles—a fraction of the 12,000 volumes I share my house with—has contributed to expanding my dream. Dear reader, you have gotten off easy. I have left out the bulk of the philosophy that lives in the world's great fiction, poetry, drama, art, cartoons, and natural sciences, as well as the 120 periodicals that come into our house, among them the *Food Insect Newsletter*, *Experimental Musical Instruments*, and *Funny Times*.

   Use this list to explore your own questions and ideas about medicine and community: browse, peruse, explore, dig in! When you come to Gesundheit and seek out the written word, I shall wear the crown of librarian.

Health and Healing

A Free Clinic Starting Out. Roanoke, VA: The Free Clinic Foundation of America, 1992.
Ader, Robert, Nicholas Cohen, and David L. Felten, eds. *Psychoneuroimmunology*, 2nd edition. SanDiego: Academic Press, 1991.
Alternative Medicine: The Definitve Guide. Puyallup, WA: Future Medicine Publishing, 1993.
Andrews, Charles. *Profit Fever: The Drive to Corporatize Health Care and How to Stop it*. Monroe, Maine: Common Courage Press, 1995
Balint, Michael, M.D. *The Doctor, His Patient and the Illness*. London: Pitman Medical, 1973.

Bauer, Jefferey. *Not What the Doctor Ordered: Reinventing Medical Care in America.* Chicago: Probus Books, 1994

Bentley, Joseph D., M.D. *The Betrayal of Health.* New York: Times Books, 1991.

Berger, John. *A Fortunate Man.* New York: Pantheon Books, 1967.

Blanton, Smiley. *Love or Perish.* New York: Simon & Schuster, 1956.

Bogdanich, Wat. *The Great White Lie: Dishonesty, Waste, and Incompetence in the Medical Community.* New York: Simon and Schuster, 1991.

Brown, E. Richard. *Rockefeller Medicine Men.* Berkeley, Ca.: University of California Press, 1979.

Broyard, Anatsle. *Intoxicated by My Illness and Other Writings on Life and Death.* New York: Clarkson Potter, 1992.

Buchanan, James. *Patient Encounters: The Experience of Disease.* Charlottesville, Va.: University of Virginia Press, 1989.

Buckman, Robert, M.D. *How to Break Bad News: A Guide for Health Care Professionals.* Baltimore: The John Hopkins University Press, 1992.

Buscaglia, Leo. *Living, Loving and Learning.* New York: Ballantine Books, 1982.

Caldicott, Helen, M.D. *If You Love this Planet: A Plan to Heal the Earth.* New York: W.W. Norton, 1992.

Califano, Joseph A., Jr. *America's Health Care Revolution.* New York: Simon & Schuster, 1986.

Callahan, Daniel. *What Kind of Life — The Limits of Medical Progress.* New York: Simon & Schuster, 1990.

Callander, Meryn G. and John W. Travis, M.D. *Wellness for Helping Professionals: Creating Compassionate Cultures.* Mill Valley, CA: Wellness Associates Publications, 1990.

Campo, Raphael. *The Poetry of Healing.* New York: W.W. Norton & Co., 1997.

Cassell, Eric J., M.D. *The Healer's Art.* Cambridge, Ma.: MIT Press, 1986.

———. *The Nature of Suffering.* New York: Oxford University Press, 1991.

———. *Talking With Patients,* Vols. 1 and 2. Cambridge, Ma.: MIT Press, 1985.

Cassell, Eric J., M.D., and Mark Siegler, M.D. *Changing Values in Medicine.* New York: University Publications of America, Inc., 1979.

Charman, Robert C., M.D. *At Risk: Can the Doctor-Patient Relationship Survive in a High-Tech World?* Dublin, NH: William L. Bauhan, 1992.

Chopra, Deepak, M.D. *Quantum Healing.* New York: Bantam Books, 1989.

Clinebell, Howard, PhD. *Well Being: A Personal Plan for Exploring and Enriching the Seven Dimensions of Life: Mind, Body, Spirit, Love, Work, Play, Earth.* San Francisco: Harper San Francisco, 1992.

Coles, Robert. *The Call of Service: A Witness to Idealism.* New York: Houghton Mifflin, 1993.

Cook, Trevor. *Samuel Hahnemann.* Wellingborough, UK: Thorsons Publishers Ltd., 1981.

Corey, Saltman Epstein. *Medicine in A Changing Society.* St. Louis: C.V. Mosby, 1977.

Coulter, Harris L. *Divided Legacy: The Conflict Between Homeopathy and the American Medical Association,* 2nd ed. Berkely: North Atlantic Books Homeopathic Educational Services, 1982.

Cousins, Norman. *Anatomy of An Illness.* New York: W. W. Norton & Co., 1979.

———. *Head First: The Biology of Hope.* New York: Dutton, 1989.

———. *The Healing Heart.* New York: W. W. Norton & Co., 1983.

————. *The Physician in Literature.* New York: Saunders Press, 1982.

Csikszentmihalyi, Mihaly. *Flow: The Psychology of Optimal Experience.* New York: Harper & Row, 1990.

Curnen, Mary, Enid Peschell, Howard Spiro, and Deborah St. James, eds. *Empathy and the Practice of Medicine.* New Haven: Yale University Press, 1993.

Dass, Ram, and Paul Gorman. *How Can I Help — Stories and Reflections on Service.* New York: Alfred A. Knopf, 1985.

Donaghue, Paul J., PhD. and Mary E. Siegel, PhD. *Sick and Tired of Feeling Sick and Tired of Feeling Sick...* New York: W.W. Norton & Co., 1992.

Dossey, Larry, M.D. *Healing Words: The Power of Prayer and the Practice of Medicine.* San Francisco, Harper San Francisco, 1993.

————. *Recovering the Soul: A Scientific and Spiritual Search.* New York: Bantam Books, 1989.

————. *Space, Time and Medicine.* Boston: New Science Library, 1982.

Drane, James F. *Becoming A Good Doctor: The Place of Virtue and Character in Medical Ethics.* Kansas City, Mo.: Sheed and Ward, 1988.

Dubos, Rene. *Mirage of Health.* New York: Doubleday Anchor Books, 1959.

————. *So Human An Animal.* New York: Charles Scribner, 1968.

Dyson, Burton, M.D., and Elizabeth Dyson. *Neighborhood Caretakers — Stories, Strategies and Tools for Healing Urban Communities.* Indianapolis: Knowledge Systems, 1989.

Dooley, Tom. *Dr. Tom Dooley's Three Great Books.* New York: Farrar, Straus & Cudahy, 1960.

Eliade, Mircea. *Shamanism.* Princeton, N.J.: Princeton University Press, 1964.

Foss, Lawrence, and Kenneth Rothaberg. *The Second Medical Revolution.* Boston: New Science Library, 1987.

Frank, Arthur W. *The Wounded Storyteller: Body, Illness, and Ethics.* Chicago: The University of Chicago Press, 1995.

Frohock, Fred M. *Healing Powers, Alternative Medicine, Spiritual Communities, and the State.* Chicago: The University of Chicago Press, 1992.

Fromm, Erich. *The Art of Loving.* New York: Harper & Row, 1956.

Galen: *Hippocrates.* Volume 10, Great Books. Chicago: Encyclopedia Britannica, 1952.

Geis, Gilbert, Paul Jesilow and Henry N. Pontell. *Prescription for Profit: How Doctors Defraud Medicaid.* Berkely: University of California Press, 1993.

Gerteis, Margret, and Susan Edgman-Levitan, et. al. *Through the Patient's Eyes.* San Francisco: Jossey-Bass Publishers, 1993

Goodnou, John C. and Gerald Musgrave. *Patient Power: Solving America's Health Care Needs.* Washington, D.C.: Cato Institute, 1992.

Gordon, James. *Manifesto for a New Medicine.* Reading, Ma.: Addison-Wesley Publishing Co., 1996.

Greenberg, Michael, M.D. *Off the Pedestal: Transforming the Business of Medicine.* Houston, Tex.: Breakthrough Publishing, 1990.

Hammerschlag, Carl A., M.D.*The Dancing Healers: A Doctor's Journey of Healing with Native Americans.* New York: Harper Collins, 1989.

————. *The Theft of the Spirit: A Journey to Spiritual Healing with Native Americans.* New York: Simon and Schuster, 1993.

Hay, Ian. *Money, Medicine, and Malpractice in American Society.* New York: Praeger, 1992.

Hertzler, Arthur. *Horse and Buggy Doctor*. New York: Harper Brothers, 1938.

Hetzel, Richard, M.D., ed. *The New Physician*. Boston: Houghton Mifflin Co., 1991.

Hilfiker, David. *Not All of Us Are Saints*. New York: Hill and Wang, 1994.

Hirshberg, Caryle and Brendan O'Regan. *Spontaneous Remission: An Annotated Bibliography*. Sausalito: Institute of Noetic Sciences, 1993.

Hunter, Kathryn Montgomery. *Doctor's Stories: The Narrative Structure of Medical Knowledge*. Princeton: Princeton University Press, 1992.

Illich, Ivan. *Medical Nemesis — The Expropriation of Health*. New York: Pantheon, 1976.

Jampolsky, Gerald G., M.D. *Love Is Letting Go of Fear*. New York: Bantam Books, 1970.

Jesdow, Paul, Henry N. Pontell, and Gilbert Geis. *Prescription for Profit: How Doctors Defraud Medicare*. Berkely: University of California Press, 1993.

Jones, James H. *Bad Blood*. New York: The Free Press, 1981.

Jonsen, Albert R. *The New Medicine and the Old Ethics*. Cambridge, Ma.: Harvard University Press, 1990.

Justice, Blair, Ph.D. *Who Gets Sick*. Los Angeles: Jeremy Tarcher, Inc., 1988.

Kassler, Jeanne, M.D. *Bitter Medicine: Greed and Chaos in American Health Care*. New York: Birch Lane Press, 1994.

Konner, Melvin. *Medicine at the Crossroads: The Crisis With Health Care*. New York: Pantheon Books, 1993.

Kaysen, Susanna. *Girl, Interrupted*. New York: Vintage Books, 1993.

Kleinman, Arthur, M.D. *The Illness Narratives*. New York: Basic Books, 1988.

Krementz, Jill. *How it Feels to Live with a Physical Disability*. New York: Simon and Schuster, 1992.

Lanctôt, Gaylaine. *The Medical Mafia: How to Get out of it Alive and Take Back Our Health and Wealth*. Morgan, Vt.: Key Inc., 1995

Lantos, John D. *Do We Still Need Doctors?* New York: Routledge, 1997.

Leebov, Wendy, Ed.D. *Service Excellence: The Customer Relations Strategy for Health Care*. Chicago: American Hospital Association Publishing, Inc., 1988.

Levoy, Gregg. *Callings: Finding and Following an Authentic Life*. New York: Harmony Books, 1997.

Lewer, Nick. *Physicians and the Peace Movement*. London: Frank Cass & Co., Ltd., 1992.

Lifton, Robert Jay. *The Protean Self: Human Resilience in an Age of Fragmentation*. New York: Basic Books, 1993.

Lipp, Martin R., M.D. *Respectful Treatment: The Human Side of Medical Care*. New York: Harper & Row, 1977.

Lowenstein, Jerome, M.D. *The Midnight Meal and other Essays about Doctors, Patients, and Medicine*. New Haven: Yale University Press, 1997.

Lown, Bernard, *The Lost Art of Healing*. Boston: Houghton Mifflin Co., 1996.

Macklin, Ruth. *Enemies of Patients: How Doctors are Losing Their Power. . . And Patients are Losing Their Rights*. New York: Oxford University Press, 1993.

Marti-Ibanez, Felix, M.D. *The Patient's Progress*. New York: M.D. Publications, 1967.

Massad, Stewart. *Doctors and Other Casualties: Stories of Life and Love Among the Healers*. New York: Warner Books, 1993.

Morone, James A. and Gary S. Belkin, ed. *The Politics of Health Care Reform: Lessons from the Past, Prospects for the Future*. Durham: Duke University Press, 1994.

Matthews, Bonnye L. *Chemical Sensitivity: A Guide to Coping with Hypersensitivity*

Syndrome, Sick Building Syndrome and Other Environmental Illness. Jefferson, NC: McFarland and Co., Inc., 1992.

McEwen, James, C. Martini, and H. Wilkins. *Participation in Health*. London: Croom Helm, 1983.

Mendelsohn, Robert S., M.D. *Confessions of a Medical Heretic*. Chicago: Contemporary Books, Inc., 1979.

Moore, Allen H., M.D. *Mustard Plasters and Printer's Ink*. New York: Exposition Press, Inc., 1959.

Morris, David B. *The Culture of Pain*. Berkeley, Ca.: University of California Press, 1991.

Moss, Ralph W. *The Cancer Industry*. New York: Paragon House, 1989.

Nichols, Joe D., M.D., and James Presley. *Please, Doctor, Do Something*. Old Greenwich, Ct.: The Devin-Adair Company, 1972.

Nolen, William, M.D. *A Surgeon's Book of Hope*. New York: Coward, McCann & Geoghan, 1980.

Noms, Richard, M.D. *The Musician's Survival Manual: A Guide to Preventing and Treating Injuries to Instrumentalists*. St. Louis: International Conference of Symphony and Opera Musicians, 1993.

Oglesby, Paul. *The Caring Physician: The Life of Dr. Francis W. Peabody*. Boston: The Francis Countway Library of Medicine in Cooperation with The Harvard Medical Alumni Association, 1991.

Osler, Sir William. *A Way of Life and Selected Writings*. New York: Dover Books, 1951.

Pagel, Walter. *Paracelsus — An Introduction To Philosophical Medicine in the Era of the Renaissance*, 2nd ed. Basel: S. Karger, 1982.

Pearse, I. H. *The Quality of Life*. Edinburgh: Scottish Academic Press, 1979.

Peck, M. Scott, M.D. *The Road Less Traveled*. New York: Simon & Schuster, 1978.

Pekkanen, John, M.D. *Doctors Talk About Themselves*. New York: Delacorte Press, 1988.

Podvoll, Edward M., M.D.*The Seduction of Madness*. New York: Harper Collins,1990.

Polk, Steven R., M.D. *The Medical Students Survival guide*. Trentland Press, 1992.

Prieto, Jorge, M.D. *Harvest of Hope*. Notre Dame, In: University of Notre Dame Press, 1989.

Reich, Warren T., ed. *Encyclopedia of Bioethics*. New York: Free Press, 1978.

Reynolds, Richard, M.D., and John Stone, M.D., eds. *On Doctoring*. New York: Simon & Schuster, 1991.

Rosenberg, Charles. *The Care of Strangers — The Rise of America's Hospital System*. New York: Basic Books, 1987.

Rodwin, Mark A. *Medicine, Money and Morals*. New York: Oxford University Press, 1993.

Schweitzer, Albert, M.D. *Albert Schweitzer: An Anthology*. Boston: Beacon Press, 1947.

Selzer, Richard. *Mortal Lessons*. New York: Simon & Schuster, 1974.

———. *Taking the World in for Repairs*. New York: William Morrow & Co., 1986.

Shames, Karilee Halo, R.N., PhD.*The Nightingale Conspiracy: Nursing Comes to Power in the 21st Century*. Staten Island: Power Publications, 1993.

Shapiro, Martin, M.D. *Getting Doctored*. Philadelphia: New Society Publishers, 1987.

Sheehan, Susan. *Is There No Place on Earth for Me?* New York: Random House, 1983.

Sherwin, Susan. *No Longer Patient: Feminist Ethics and Health Care*. Philadelphia: Temple University Press, 1992.

Shorter, Edward. *Doctors and Their Patients*. New Brunswick, N.J.: Transaction Publishers, 1991.

Siegel, Bernie S., M.D. *Peace, Love & Healing.* New York: Harper & Row, 1989.

———. *Love, Medicine & Miracles.* New York: Harper & Row, 1986.

Smith, John M., M.D. *Women and Doctors: A Physician's Explosive Account of Women's Medical Treatment—and Mistreatment—in America Today and What You Can do About It.* New York: The Atlantic Monthly Press, 1992.

Sontag, Susan. *Illness as Metaphor.* New York: Random House, 1979.

Starr, Paul. *The Social Transformation of American Medicine.* New York: Basic Books, 1982.

Stevens, Rosemary. *In Sickness and In Wealth.* New York: Basic Books, 1989.

Stratton, Owen Tully. *Medicine Many.* London: University of Oklahoma Press, 1989.

Thomas, Lewis. *The Fragile Species.* New York: Charles Scribner's Sons, 1992.

———. *Late Night Thoughts on Listening to Mahler's Ninth Symphony.* New York: Viking Press, 1983.

———. *The Lives of A Cell.* New York: Bantam Books, 1975.

———. *The Medusa and the Snail.* New York: Viking Press, 1978.

———. *The Youngest Science.* New York: Bantam Books, 1984.

Thomasma, David. *Human Life in the Balance.* Louisville, Ky.: Westminster / John Knox Press, 1990.

Thompson, John, and Grace Goldin. *The Hospital: A Social and Architectural History.* New Haven, Ct: Yale University Press, 1975

Weil, Andrew, M.D. *Health and Healing.* Boston: Houghton Mifflin Co., 1983.

Weiss, Raymond L., and Charles E. Butterworth. *Ethical Writings of Maimonides.* New York: NYU Press, 1975.

Werner, David, and David Sanders. *The Politics of Primary Health Care and Child Survival.* Palo Alto, Ca.: Healthwrights, 1997.

Williamson, G. Scott, and Innes H. Pearse. *Science, Synthesis and Sanity.* Edinburgh: Scottish Academic Press, 1980.

Wohl, Stanley, M.D. *The Medical Industrial Complex.* New York: Harmony Books, 1984.

Wolf, Stewart, and John G. Bruhn. *The Power of Clan: The Influence of Human Relations on Heart Disease.* New Brunswick: Transaction Publishers, 1993.

Physicians' Values

Alda, Alan. "Alan Alda's Prescription for Doctors." *Good Housekeeping* October 1979.

Barber, Bernard, Ph.D. "Compassion in Medicine: Toward New Definitions and New Institutions." *Seminars in Medicine of Beth Israel Hospital* 295, no. 17 (1976).

Bowen, Otis R., M.D. "Shattuck Lecture—What Is Quality Care?" *New England Journal of Medicine* 316, no. 25 (1987).

Boyle, Joseph F., M.D. "Should We Learn to Say No?" *JAMA* 252, no. 6 (1984).

Bunker, John P. "When Doctors Disagree." *New York Review of Books* April 25, 1985.

Burnum, John, M.D. "Medical Practice a la Mode." *New England Journal of Medicine* 317, no. 19 (1987).

Cassel, Eric J., M.D. "The Nature of Suffering and the Goals of Medicine." *New England Journal of Medicine* 306, no. 11 (1982).

Cohen, Carl I., M.D., and Ellen J. Cohen, Ph.D. "Health Education, Panacea, Pernicious or Pointless." *New England Journal of Medicine* 299, no. 13 (1978).

Coles, Robert, M.D., "The Doctor Is In." *Common Cause Magazine* May / June 1988, pp. 25–29.

Corboy, John, M.D. "Don't Forget the Magic." *American Medical News* June 25—July 2, 1982.

Council of Medical Service. "Quality of Care." *JAMA* 256, no. 8 (1986).

Coury, John Jr., M.D. "Physicians' Fundamental Responsibility." *JAMA* 256, no. 8 (1986).

Darrow, Gregory R., M.D. "If Your Daughter Survives, Doctor, She's Going to be a Gork." *Medical Economics* July 25, 1983.

Deckert, Gordon, M.D. "Urges Physicians to Play More; Avoid Turning Play into Work." *Pediatric News* 20, no. 3 (1986).

Dimsky, S. Edwards, M.D. "Why Not Share the Secrets of Good Health?" *JAMA* 249, no. 23 (1983).

Dirck, John H., M.D. "Sir Thomas Browne (1605–1682)." *JAMA* 248, no. 15 (1982).

Edwards, W. Sterling, M.D. "In Retirement, A Doctor Learns to Truly Listen." *AMA News* October 20, 1989, p. 43.

Gabbard, Glen, M.D. "The Role of Compulsiveness in the Normal Physician." *JAMA* 254, no. 20 (1985).

Guzi, Samuel B., M.D. "Can the Practice of Medicine be Fun for a Lifetime?" *JAMA* 241, no. 19 (1979).

Hilfiker, David, M.D. "Unconscious on a Corner." *JAMA* 258, no. 21 (1987).

Horn, Carole, M.D. "There's Art in Being a Doctor." *Washington Post* October 28, 1984.

Hyman, David. "Fraud and Abuse, Setting Limits on Physicians' Entrepreneurship." *New England Journal of Medicine* 320, no. 19 (1989).

Jansen, Albert R., Ph.D. "Watching the Doctor." *New England Journal of Medicine* 308, no. 25 (1983).

Jirka, Frank J. Jr., M.D. "Travelling New Streets." *JAMA* 250, no. 11 (1983).

John Paul II, Pope. "The Physician and the Rights of Mankind." *JAMA* 251, no. 8 (1984).

Kass, Leon R., M.D., Ph. D. "Ethical Dilemmas in the Care of the Ill." *JAMA* 244, no. 16 (1980).

Korok, Milan. "From Patient Advocate to Gatekeeper." Symposium on Health Care. *American Medical News* April 4, 1986.

Levinson, Wendy, M.D. "Coping with Fallibility." *JAMA* 261, no. 15 (1989).

Marzuk, Peter, M.D. "When the Patient is a Physician." *New England Journal of Medicine* 317, no. 22 (1987).

Mathiasen, Helle, Ph.D., and Joseph Alpert, M.D. "Medicine and Literature in the Medical Curriculum." *JAMA* 244, no. 13 (1980).

McClenahan, John L., M.D. "An Apple for the Teacher." *MD* September 1982 p. 13.

McCue, Jack D., M.D. "The Effects of Stress on Physicians and Their Medical Practice." *New England Journal of Medicine* 306, no. 8 (1982).

Nicholson, Ian, "Sometimes, Physicians Need to Take the Time to Care." *AMA News* November 18, 1988, p. 27.

O'Donnell, Walter E., M.D. "Why 'Me First' is Ruining Medicine." *Medical Economics* September 27, 1982.

Osmond, Humphrey, MCRP., F.R.C. Psych., F.R.C.P. "God and the Doctor." *New England Journal of Medicine* 302, no. 10 (1980).

Pellegrino, Edmond, M.D. "Altruism, Self-Interest and Medical Ethics." *JAMA* 258, no. 14 (1987).

Radetsky, Michael, M.D. "Recapturing the Spirit in Medicine." *New England Journal of Medicine* 298, no. 20 (1978).

Risse, Guenter B., M.D. "Whither Healing." *MD*, February 1979.

Rodwin, Marc, M.D. "Physicians' Conflict of Interest." *New England Journal of Medicine* 259, no. 22 (1989).

Southgate, M. Therese, M.D. "Simple Gifts." *JAMA* 245, no. 17 (1981).

Steptoe, Sonja."Dispirited Doctors, Hassles and Red Tape Destroy Joy of the Job for Many Physicians." *Wall Street Journal* April 10, 1987.

Tanay, Emanuel, M.D. "Our Next Endangered Species: The Dedicated Doctor." *Medical Economics* December 7, 1981.

Watts, Malcolm, M.D. "Medicine Has Room for Both 'Breeds' of M.D.s." *AMA News* August 11, 1989, p. 28.

Weed, Lawrence L., M.D. "Physicians of the Future." *New England Journal of Medicine* 304, no. 15 (1981).

Wynen, Andre, M.D. "The World Medical Association and Medical Ethics." *JAMA* 251, no. 8 (1984).

Zinn, William, M.D. "Doctors Have Feelings Too." *New England Journal of Medicine* 259, no. 22 (1988).

Physician Education

Association of American Medical Colleges. "Physicians for the Twenty-First Century." *The GPEP Report*, 1984.

Bickel, Janet. "Human Values Teaching Programs in the Clinical Education of Medical Students." *Journal of Medical Education* May 1987, Vol. 62.

Billings, J. Andrew, M.D., et al. "A Seminar in Plain Doctoring." *Journal of Medical Education* November 1985, Vol. 60.

Brailer, David, M.D. and David Nash, M.D. "Uncertainty and the Future of Young Physicians." *JAMA* 256, no. 24 (1986).

Brauer, Arlette. "Humanizing Medicine." *MD* October 1982.

Bressler, David. "Notes From Overground." *JAMA* 245, no. 16 (1981).

Brown, Sue. "Why New Doctors Aren't Ready for Practice." *Medical Economics* July 25, 1983.

Clark, David, et al. "Vicissitudes of Depressed Mood During Four Years of Medical School." *JAMA* 260, no. 17 (1988).

Cohen, Mark L., M.D. "Uncertainty Rounds." *JAMA* 250, no. 13 (1983).

Colford, John Jr., M.D. "The Ravelled Sleeve of Care, Managing the Stresses of Residency Training." *JAMA* 261, no. 6 (1989).

Council on Long Range Planning and Development of AMA. "Health Care in Transition, Consequences for Young Physicians." *JAMA* 256, no. 24 (1986).

"Disaffection of Doctors Is Discouraging Medical Students and Potential Ones." *Wall Street Journal* April 10, 1987.

Dubovsky, Steven L., M.D. and Robert W. Schriu, M.D. "The Mystique of Medical Training." *JAMA* 250, no. 22 (1983).

Eichna, Ludwig W., M.D. "Medical School Education, 1975–1979." *New England Journal of Medicine* 303, no. 13 (1980).

Glick, Seymour M., M.D. "Humanistic Medicine in a Modern Age." *New England Journal of Medicine* 304, no. 17 (1981).

Henry, John Bernard, M.D. "Dean's Welcome Remarks to the Class of 1986." *JAMA* 249, no. 12 (1983).

Johnson, Roger S., Ph.D. "Confront 'Dehumanization' Problem." *Medical Tribune* April 4, 1984.

Kapelman, Loretta, Ph.D. "Cynicism Among Medical Students." *JAMA* 250, no. 15 (1983).

McCue, Jack D., M.D. "The Distress of Internship." *New England Journal of Medicine* 312, no. 7 (1985).

Pence, Gregory E., Ph.D. "Medical Students Need Perspective, Hope." *American Medical News* November 7, 1986.

Perersdorf, Robert G., M.D. "Is the Establishment Defensible." *New England Journal of Medicine* 309, no. 17 (1983).

Rosenberg, Donna A., M.D. and Henry K. Silver, M.D. "Medical Student Abuse." *JAMA* 251, no. 6 (1984).

Schroeder, Steven, M.D. "Academic Medicine as a Public Trust." *JAMA* 262, no. 6 (1989).

Tasteson, D.C., M.D. "Learning in Medicine." *New England Journal of Medicine* September 27, 1979.

Thomas, Lewis. "What Doctors Don't Know." *New York Review of Books* September 24, 1987, p. 6.

Weissmann, Gerald, "A Slap of the Tail: Reading Medical Humanities." *Hospital Practice* June 15, 1988.

Malpractice

Bowen, Otis R., M.D. "Shattuck Lecture—What Is Quality Care?" *New England Journal of Medicine* 316, no. 25 (1987).

Bryan, Charles, M.D. "A M.D. Remembers a Malpractice Suit: 'I've Been There.'" *AMA News* March 17, 1989, p. 55.

Bunker, John P. "When Doctors Disagree." *New York Review of Books* April 25, 1985.

Burnum, John, M.D. "Medical Practice a la Mode." *New England Journal of Medicine* 317, no. 19 (1987).

Challones, David, M.D., et al. "Effects of Liability Crisis on the Academic Health Center." *New England Journal of Medicine* 319, no. 24 (1988).

Cohen, Jon. "Dr. Quixote, Gabor Laufer, M.D., Waged a Private Battle for Tort Reform." *AMA News* March 17, 1989, p. 55.

Council of Medical Service. "Quality of Care." *JAMA* 256, no. 8 (1986).

Coury, John Jr., M.D. "Physicians' Fundamental Responsibility." *JAMA* 256, no. 8 (1986).

Deckert, Gordon, M.D. "Urges Physicians to Play More; Avoid Turning Play into Work." *Pediatric News* 20, no. 3 (1986).

"Fear of Suits Affecting Practice of Medicine." Editorial. *AMA News* June 30, 1989, p. 15.

Gabbard, Glen, M.D. "The Role of Compulsiveness in the Normal Physician." *JAMA* 254, no. 20 (1985).

Goldberg, Joel. "The Great Doctor Revolt." *Medical Economics* July 3, 1989.

Hiatt, Howard, M.D., et al. "A Study of Medical Injury and Medical Malpractice." *New England Journal of Medicine* 321, no. 7 (1989).

Hilfiker, David, M.D. "Unconscious on a Corner." *JAMA* 258, no. 21 (1987).

Horn, Carole, M.D. "There's Art in Being a Doctor." *Washington Post* October 28, 1984.

Korcok, Milan. "From Patient Advocate to Gatekeeper." Symposium on Health Care. *American Medical News* April 4, 1986.

Kubetin, Sally K. "Pediatricians Told To Do More To Confront Crisis in Liability." *Pediatric News* January 1988, p. 2.

Marzuk, Peter, M.D. "When the Patient Is a Physician." *New England Journal of Medicine* 317, no. 22 (1987).

Moskowitz, R., M.D. "Some Thoughts on the Malpractice Crisis." *British Homeopathic Journal* January 1988, p. 77.

Paris, Joseph, M.D. "Current System Will Not Solve Malpractice Crisis." *AMA News* January 8, 1988, p. 40.

Paxton, Harry. "Just How Heavy is the Burden of Malpractice Premiums." *Medical Economy* January 16, 1989.

Pellegrino, Edmond, M.D. "Altruism, Self-Interest and Medical Ethics." *JAMA* 258, no. 14 (1987).

Schwartz, William, M.D., et al. "Physicians Who have Lost Their Malpractice Insurance." *JAMA* 262, no. 10 (1989).

"Special Issue on Malpractice." *Medical Economics* April 18, 1989.

Steptoe, Sonja. "Dispirited Doctors, Hassles and Red Tape Destroy Joy of the Job for Many Physicians." *Wall Street Journal* April 10, 1987.

Doctor-Patient Relationship

Adelson, Bernard H., M.D. "Ethical Decisions in Medicine." *MD* February 1983.

Ansell, David, M.D., and Robert Schiff, M.D. "Patient Dumping." *JAMA* 257, no. 11 (1987).

Cohn, Victor. "Putting the Patients in Charge." *Washington Post* February 26, 1986.

Conger, Charles, M.D. "Now I Know Why Patients Sometimes Scream at Doctors." *Medical Economics* January 16, 1989.

Council on Long Range Planning, AMA House of Delegates. "Survey: M.D.'s Public Image Going Down." *American Medical News* June 28, 1985.

Cousins, Norman. "How Patients Appraise Physicians." *New England Journal of Medicine* 313, no. 22 (1985).

———. "Intangibles in Medicine: An Attempt at Balancing Perspectives." *JAMA* September 23, 1988, p. 26.

———. "The Physician as Communicator." *JAMA* 248, no. 5 (1982).

———. "Unacceptable Pressures on the Physician." *JAMA* 252, no. 3 (1984).

Davidson, Charles, M.D. "Respecting the Autonomy of Competent Patients." *New England Journal of Medicine* 310, no. 17 (1984).

"Deterioration of the Physician/Patient Relationship." Commentary. *American Medical News* October 23, 1987.

Dolan, Barbara, et al. "Doctors and Patients: Image vs. Reality." *Time* July 31, 1989.

Egeer, Ross L., M.D. "I Make My Patients Be Their Own Doctors." *Medical Economics* June 12, 1978.

Gorlin, Richard, M.D., and Howard D. Zucker, M.D. "Physician's Reaction to Patients." *New England Journal of Medicine* 308, no. 18 (1983).

Hardy, Clyde T. Jr. "What Ever Happened to Dr. Nice Guy." *Medical Economics* February 3, 1986.

Hilfiker, David, M.D. "Facing Our Mistakes." *New England Journal of Medicine* 310, no. 2 (1984).

Hogness, John R., M.D. "What About the Patient?" *New England Journal of Medicine* 313, no. 11 (1985).

Jacoby, M.G., M.B., B.S. "A Father's Letter to a New Intern." *JAMA* 245, no. 10 (1981).

Kassiru, Jerome P., M.D. "Adding Insult to Injury." *New England Journal of Medicine* 308, no. 15 (1983).

Lesser, Gershon, M.D. "Don't Lose Sight of the Human Factor in Patient Care." *AMA News* September 9, 1988, p. 25.

Marzuk, Peter, M.D. "The Right Kind of Patemalism." *New England Journal of Medicine* 313, no. 23 (1985).

Mindell, Benjamin. "Patients Rate Friendliness High Among Physician Traits." *AMA News* February 19, 1988, p. 13.

Neumann, Hans, M.D. "Why Have We Stopped Comforting Patients?" *Medical Economics* June 22, 1987.

Perrone, Janice. "Dr. Davis Urges Physicians: Give a 'Tithe of Your Time'." *AMA News* July 8, 1988, p. 1.

Pinkney, Deborah. "Manpower Crisis." *American Medical News* November 20, 1987.

Quill, Timothy E., M.D. "Patient-Centered Medicine: Increasing Patient Responsibility." *Hospital Practice* November 30, 1985.

Sackler, Arthur M., M.D. "The Doctor Is One of the Patient's Best Friends." *Medical Tribune* June 29, 1983.

Sheldon, Mark, Ph.D. "Truth Telling in Medicine." *JAMA* 247, no. 5 (1982).

Skelly, Flora. "Good M.D.–Patient Relationship Linked to Good Outcome." *AMA News* June 9, 1989, p. 3.

Strull, William M., M.D. et al. "Do Patients Want to Participate in Medical Decision Making?" *JAMA* 292, no. 21 (1984).

Taylor, Flora. "When You and Your Partner The Doctor Talk About Diagnosis." *FDA Consumer* November 1979.

Taylor, Richard, M.D. "Don't Forget Personal in Midst of Technology." *AMA News* May 13, 1988, p. 37.

Teich, Judith. "Primary Care." *JAMA* 259, no. 17 (1988).

Waldron, Vincent D., M.D. "What To Do When Your Patient Isn't Going to Get Better." *Medical Economics* December 20, 1982.

Wassersug, Joseph D., M.D. "What You'll Never Learn Unless You Make House Calls." *Medical Economics* July 22, 1985.

Watts, Malcolm, M.D. "Are Frustrated, Angry M.D.s Good for Health Care?" *AMA News* September 23, 1988, p. 26.

Weaver, James, M.D. "Share Uncertainties of Medical Therapy with Patients." *AMA News* September 9, 1988, p. 32.

Health Care Delivery

"Access to Care and the Evolutions of Corporate, For-Profit Medicine." *New England Journal of Medicine* 311, no. 14 (1984).

Ansell, David, M.D. and Robert Schiff, M.D. "Patient Dumping." *JAMA* 257, no. 11 (1987).

Armitage, Karen J., M.D., et al. "Response of Physicians to Medical Complaints in Men and Women." *JAMA* 241, no. 20 (1979).

Atkins, Charles. "Dollars Must Not Take Precedence Over Care." *AMA News* September 8, 1989, p. 32.

Bezold, Clement. "Health Care in the U.S." *The Futurist* August, 1982.

Bortz , Walter M. II, M.D. "Disuse and Aging." *JAMA* 248, no. 10 (1982).

Califano, Joseph, M.D. "Billions Blown on Health." *New York Times* April 4, 1989.

Castro, Janice. "Critical Condition: Defying All Expectations, Health Costs Continue to Soar." *TIME* February 1,1988, pp. 42–43.

Cohn, Victor. "Caring and Cash Come into Conflict." *Washington Post Health* September 27, 1989, p. 11.

———. "Putting the Patients in Charge." *The Washington Post* February 26, 1986.

"Commercialization Said to Threaten M.D.–Patient Trust." Editorial, *Pediatric News* 22, no. 1 (1988).

Couch, Nathan P., M.D., et al. "The High Cost of Low-Frequency Events." *New England Journal of Medicine* 304, no. 11 (1981).

Council on Long Range Planning, AMA House of Delegates. "Survey: M.D.'s Public Image Going Down." *American Medical News* June 28, 1985.

Cousins, Norman. "How Patients Appraise Physicians." *New England Journal of Medicine* 313, no. 22 (1985).

Crawshaw, Ruth, M.D. "Has the Machine Become the Physician?" *JAMA* 250, no. 4 (1983).

Crile, George Jr. "High-Tech Medicine We Can't Afford." *Washington Post* July 31, 1983.

Davis, James E., M.D. "National Initiatives for Care of the Medical Needy." *JAMA* 259, no. 21 (1988).

DeBakey, Michael E., M.D. "Caring Is What Counts." *American Medical News* May 29, 1981.

Del Guercio, Louis R. M., M.D. "Hippocrates Would be Ashamed of Us—Rightfully So!" *Medical Economics* May 15, 1978.

"Deterioration of the Physician / Patient Relationship." Commentary. *American Medical News* October 23, 1987.

Drummond, Hugh, M.D. "Your Health at Too High a Premium." *Mother Jones* May, 1977.

Ehrbar, A.F. "A Radical Prescription for Medical Care." *Fortune* February 1977.

Enthoven, Alain C., Ph.D. "Consumer-Choice Health Plan." *New England Journal of Medicine* 298, no. 12 (1978).

Evans, Robert G. "Controlling Health Expenditures, the Guardian Reality." *New England Journal of Medicine* 320, no. 9 (1989).

Ginzberg, Eli, Ph.D. "The Grand Illusion of Competition in Health Care." *JAMA* 249, no. 10 (1983).

———. "Medical Care for the Poor: No Magic Bullets." *JAMA* 259, no. 21 (1988).

Gould, Jeffrey, M.D. "Socioeconomic Differences with Rate of C-Section." *New England Journal of Medicine* 321, no. 4 (1989).

Goumet, Gerald, M.D. "Health Care Rationing through Rationing." *New England Journal of Medicine* 321, no. 9 (1989).

Gray, James. "How Serious Are Employers About Cutting Health Costs? Very." *Medical Economics* October 16, 1989.

Hancock, Trevor. "Beyond Health Care." *The Futurist* August 1982.

Hardy, Clyde T. Jr. "What Ever Happened to Dr. Nice Guy?" *Medical Economics* February 3, 1986.

"Health Cost: What Limit?" *Time* May 28, 1979.

Hellman, Alan, M.D., et. al. "How Do Financial Incentives Affect Physician's Clinical Decisions and the Financial Performance of Health Maintenance Organizations?" *New England Journal of Medicine* 321, no. 2 (1989).

Hogness, John R., M.D. "What About the Patient?" *New England Journal of Medicine* 313, no. 11 (1985).

Iglehart, John K., "Payment of Physicians Under Medicare." *New England Journal of Medicine* 318, no. 13 (1988).

———. "The Debate over Physician Ownership of Health Care Facilities." *New England Journal of Medicine* 321, no. 3 (1989).

Kassirer, Jerome, M.D. "Our Stubborn Quest for Diagnostic Certainty." *New England Journal of Medicine* 320, no. 22 (1989).

Kimball, Merit. "AMA Goes to War Against Limits on Doctor Payments." *Health Week* July 17, 1989, p. 9.

———. "Doctors Who Own Labs Order More Costly Tests." *Health Week* June 12, 1989, p.6.

Kinzer, David. "The Decline and Fall of Deregulation." *New England Journal of Medicine* 318, no. 2 (1988).

Kirchner, Merian. "How Much Trouble Is your Hospital in?" *Medical Economics*, December 19, 1988.

Leaf, Alexander, M.D. "Cost Effectiveness as a Criterion for Medicare Coverage." *New England Journal of Medicine* 321, no. 13 (1989).

Linzer, Mark, M.D. "Doing What 'Needs' to Be Done." *New England Journal of Medicine* 310, no. 7 (1984).

Madison, Donald L., M.D. "The Case for Community-Oriented Primary Care." *JAMA* 249, no. 10 (1983).

Marzuk, Peter, M.D. "The Right Kind of Paternalism." *New England Journal of Medicine* 313, no. 23 (1985).

McClenohan, John L., M.D. "On Going to the Doctor." *MD* September 1980.

Morreim, E. Haavi. "Conflicts of Interest—Profits and Problems in Physician Referrals," *JAMA* 262, no. 3 (1989).

Moxley, John III, M.D. "Is the Care of the Chronically Ill a Medical Prerogative?" *New England Journal of Medicine* 310, no. 3 (1984).

Neumann, Hans, M.D. "Why Have We Stopped Comforting Patients?" *Medical Economics* June 22, 1987.

Nowak, Barbara W. "Marketing Medicine to Today's Consumer." *JAMA* 242, no. 22 (1979).
Nuzzo, Roy, M.D. "Medicaid Inequities." *Infectious Diseases of Children* June 1989, p. 3.
Pinkney, Deborah S., "Hospitals Closures Up! Few MDS Patients." *AMA News* May 19, 1989, p. 1.
———. "Manpower Crisis." *American Medical News* November 20, 1987.
———. "Patient's Access to Hospital Care Eroding." *AMA News* February 19, 1988, p. 11.
Plumeri, Peter P., DO, JD, LLM. "Finally . . . A Treatable Illness." *JAMA* 250, no. 10 (1983).
Quill, Timothy E., M.D. "Patient-Centered Medicine: Increasing Patient Responsibility." *Hospital Practice* November 30, 1985.
Reagan, Michael. "Health Care Rationing." *New England Journal of Medicine* 319, no. 12 (1988).
Relman, Arnold, M.D. "The National Leadership Commission's Health Care Plan." *New England Journal of Medicine* 320, no. 5 (1989).
———. "Salaried Physicians and Economic Incentives." *New England Journal of Medicine* 319, p. 12 (1988).
Saltzman, Robert L., M.D. "Time to Return to Basics." *American Medical News* September 28, 1984.
Samuelson, Robert J. "Why Medical Costs Keep Soaring." *Washington Post* November 30, 1988, p. A23.
Saward, Ernest, M.D. "Competition and Health Care." *New England Journal of Medicine* 306, no. 15 (1982).
———. "Reflections on Change in Medical Practice." *JAMA* 250, no. 20 (1983).
Scheier, Ronni. "Learning to Practice the Business of Medicine." *AMA News* January 20, 1989 p. 41.
Schneider, Edward, M.D. "Options to Control the Rising Health Care Costs of Older Americans." *JAMA* 261, no. 6 (1989).
Schramn, Carl J., Ph.D. "Can We Solve the Hospital-Cost Problem in Our Democracy?" *New England Journal of Medicine* 311, no. 11 (1984).
Scoltoch, John, M.D. "Look What the Profit Motive Is Doing to Us Doctors!" *Medical Economics* February 6, 1978.
Siegel, Mark, M.D. "A Physician's Perspective on a Right to Health Care." *JAMA* 244, no. 14 (1980).
Snyder, Richard D. "Health Hazard Appraisal." *The Futurist* August 1982.
Steel, Knight, M.D., et al. "Iatrogenic Illness on a General Medical Service at a University Hospital." *New England Journal of Medicine* 304, no. 11 (1981) .
Strull, William M., M.D., et al. "Do Patients Want to Participate in Medical Decision Making?" *JAMA* 292, no. 21 (1984).
Todd, James S., M.D. "It Is Time for Universal Access, Not Universal Insurance." *New England Journal of Medicine* 321, no. 1 (1989).
Trunet, Patrick, M.D. "The Role of Iatrogenic Disease in Admissions to Intensive Care." *JAMA* 244, no. 23 (1980).
Walsh, H. Gilbert, M.D., et al. "Dealing with Limited Resources." *New England Journal of Medicine* 310, no. 3 (1988).
Wassersug, Joseph D., M.D. "What You'll Never Learn Unless You Make House Calls." *Medical Economics* July 22, 1985.
Watts, Malcolm, M.D. "The Dilemma of Favoring Dollars over Doctoring." *AMA News* November 18, 1988, p. 25.

————. "We're Missing the Point in Cutting Health Costs." *AMA News* 319, p. 27 (1988).
Woolhandler, Steffie, M.D., et al. "A National Health Program: Northern Light at the End of the Tunnel." *JAMA* 262, no. 15 (1989).

Perspectives on Health and Healing

Barsky, Arthur. "The Paradox of Health." *New England Journal of Medicine* 318, no. 7 (1988).
Berwick, Donald, M.D. "Continuous Improvement as An Ideal in Health Care." *New England Journal of Medicine* 320, no. 1 (1989).
Boisaubin, Eugene V., M.D. "A Barefoot Physician." *JAMA* 249, no. 1 (1983).
Close, William, M.D. "Real Medicine, As Practiced in the 'Boonies'." *AMA News* September 9, 1988, p. 48.
Cranshaw, Ralph, M.D. "A Lesson from Chinese Medicine." *JAMA* November 17, 1978.
Donabedian, Avedis, M.D. "The Quality of Care—How Can It Be Assessed?" *JAMA* 260, no. 12 (1988).
French, Kimberly. "Health-Politics Connection Exposed in New York." *Whole Life Times* January/February, 1983.
Gillick, Muriel B., M.D. "Common-Sense Models of Health and Disease." 313, no. 11 (1985).
Godden, J.O., M.D. "The Role of Belief in the Healing Process." Conference on Continuing Education, McMaster University Medical School. February 3, 1983.
Gorden, James S., M.D. "Holistic Medicine: Toward a New Medical Model." *Journal of Clinical Psychiatry* 42 vol. 3 (1981).
Harris, T. George. "Beyond Self." *American Health* March 1988, pp. 51–71.
Iotta, Dennis, M.D. "Wellness Put My Practice in Shape." *Medical Economics* 220, no. 13 (1988).
Martin, Morgan, M.D. "Native American Medicine." *JAMA* 245, no. 2 (1981).
Meyer, Harris. "Dr. Nelson Urges M.D.s to Stress Humanism." *AMA News* July 1989.
Muna, Walinjam F.T., M.D. "How I Encountered the Sophisticated Traditional Healer." *JAMA* 246, no. 22 (1981).
Nelson, Alan, M.D. "Humanism and the Art of Medicine, Our Commitment to Care." *JAMA* 262, no. 9 (1989).
Pedoisky, M. Lawrence, M.D. "Is Holistic Medicine Filling a Gap We've Created?" *Medical Economics* December 11, 1978.
"Psychiatric Sanctuary." *MD* July 1979.
Seliger, Susan. "Stop Killing Yourself." *Washingtonian* September 1978.
Shapiro, Edith, M.D. "Medical Profession Needs to Regain Its Good Manners." *AMA News*, August 18, 1989, p. 31.
Skelly, Flora. "Beyond Conventional Therapy." *AMA News* November 17, 1989, p. 37.
Steffen, Grant, M.D. "Quality Medical Care." *JAMA* 260, no. 1 (1988).
Wanzer, Sidney, M.D., et al. "The Physician's Responsibility Toward Hopelessly Ill Patients." *New England Journal of Medicine* March 30, 1989.
Watts, Malcolm, M.D. "M.D.s Have Responsibility to Cure Society's Ills." *AMA News*, Jan. 13, 1989, p. 28.

Humor and Health

Baudelaire, Charles. "The Essence of Laughter," in *Essays*. New York: Meridian Books, 1956.

Bergson, H. *Laughter. An Essay on the Meaning of the Comic.* New York: Macmillan, 1911.

Berk, Lee S., et. al. "Neuroendocrine and Stress Hormone Changes During Mirthful Laughter." The American Journal of the Medical Sciences, Vol. 296, No. 7, December 1989.

Beyondananda, Swami. *When You See a Sacred Cow . . . Milk It For All It's Worth.* Lower Lake, CA: Aslan Publishing, 1993.

Blair, W. "What's Funny About Doctors." *Perspectives in Biology and Medicine*, 1977.

Blumenfeld, E., and L. Alpern. *The Smile Connection.* Englewood Cliffs, N.J.: Prentice Hall, 1986.

Bokun, Branko. *Humour Therapy.* London: Vita Books, 1986.

Boston, R. *An Anatomy of Laughter.* London: Collins, 1974.

Boxman, Karyn, RN. "Humor in Therapy for the Mentally Ill." Journal of Psychosocial Nursing, Vol. 29, No. 12, 1991.

Burton, Robert. *The Anatomy of Melancholy.* New York: Tudor Publishing Co., 1927.

Chapman, A. J., and H. C. Foot. eds. *It's A Funny Thing, Humor.* International Conference on Humor and Laughter. Oxford: Pergamon Press, 1976.

Coser, R. L. "Some Social Functions of Laughter: A Study of Humor in a Hospital Setting." *Human Relations*, 1959.

Cousins, Norman. *Anatomy of An Illness.* New York: W. W. Norton & Co., 1979.

Dana, Bill, and Laurence, Peter. *The Laughter Prescription.* New York: Ballantine, 1982.

Dearborn, G. V. N. "The Nature of the Smile and the Laugh." *Science*, 1900.

Euck, John J., Elizabeth Forter, Alvin Whitley, eds. *The Comic in Theory and Practice.* New York: Appleton-Century-Crofts, 1960.

Fairbanks, Douglas. *Laugh and Live.* New York: Britton Publishing Co., 1917.

Feibleman, James. *In Praise of Comedy.* New York: Horizon Press, 1970.

Freud, Sigmund. *Jokes and Their Relationship to the Unconscious.* New York: W.W. Norton & Co., 1964.

Fry, W. F., Jr., *Sweet Madness: A Study of Humor.* Palo Alto, Ca.: Pacific Books, 1963.

Fry, W. F., Jr., M.D. *Make 'Em Laugh.* Palo Alto: Science and Behavior Books, 1975.

Fry, W. F., Jr., and C. Rader. "The Respiratory Components of Mirthful Laughter." *Journal of Biological Psychology*, 1977.

Fry, W.F., Jr., M.D. and Waleed A. Salameh PhD., eds. *Advances in Humor and Psychology.* Sarasota: Professional Resource Press, 1993.

Gaberson, Kathleen B., RN. "The Effect of Humorous Disfunction on Preoperative Anxiety."AORN Journal, Vol. 54, No. 6, December 1991.

Glodstein, Jefferey H. and Paul McGhee, eds. *Handbook of Humor Research.* Basic Issues Vol. 1 and Applied Studies Vol. 2. New York: Springer-Verlag, 1983.

Goodheart, Annette. *Laughter Therapy.* Santa Barbara: Less Stress Press, 1994.

Grotjahn, M. *Beyond Laughter.* New York: McGraw-Hill, 1956.

Hageseth, Christian, III, M.D. *A Laughing Place.* Ft. Collins, Co.: Berwick Publishing Co., 1988.

Haller, Bernard and Rita Zarai. *Rire c'est la Santé*. Geneva: Éditions Soleil, 1986.

Harlow, H. F. "The Anatomy of Humor." *Impact of Science on Society*, 1969.

Hassett, J., and G. E. Schwartz. "Why Can't People Take Humor Seriously?" *New York Times Magazine*, February, 1977.

The Healing Power of Laughter and Play: Uses of Humor in the Healing Arts. Twelve tapes. P.O. Box 94305. Portola Valley, Ca.: IAHB, Inc., 1983.

Holden, Robert. *Laughter the Best Medicine*. London: Thorsons, 1993.

Holland, Norman. *Laughing: The Psychology of Humor*. New York: Cornell University Press, 1982.

Joubert, Laurent. *Treatise on Laughter*. Birmingham, Ala.: University of Alabama Press, 1970.

Keller, Dan. *Humor as Therapy*. Wau Watosh, Wi.: Med-Psych Publications, 1984.

Klein, Allen. *The Healing Power of Humor*. Los Angeles: Jeremy Tarcher, 1989.

Koestler, A. *The Act of Creation*. New York: Macmillan, 1964.

Levine, J. "Humor as a Form of Therapy" in *It's A Funny Thing, Humor*, ed. by A. J. Chapman and H. C. Foot. Oxford: Pergamon Press, 1976.

McConnell, J. "Confessions of a Scientific Humorist." *Impact of Science on Society*, 1969.

McHale, Maryellen, RN. "Getting the Joke: Interpreting Humor in Group Therapy." Journal of Psychological Nursing, Vol. 27, No. 9, 1989.

Metcalf, C.W. and Roma Felible. *Lighten Up*. Reading, MA: Addison-Wesley Publishing Co., 1992.

Mind, H. "The Use and Abuse of Humor in Psychotherapy" in *Humor and Laughter: Theory, Research and Application*, ed. by A. J. Chapman and H. C. Foot. New York: John Wiley & Sons, 1976.

Mindess, Harvey, et al., eds. *The Antioch Humor Test*. New York: Avon, 1985.

———. "Laughter and Humor in Medical Practice." *Behavioral Medicine*, 1979.

Moody, R. A., Jr. *Laugh After Laugh: The Healing Power of Humor*. Jacksonville, Fl.: Headwaters Press, 1978.

Paskind, H. A. "Effect of Laughter on Muscle Tone." *Archives of Neurology and Psychiatry*, 1932.

Pasquali, Elaine Anne, PhD. "Learning to Laugh: Humor as Therapy." Journal of Psychological Nursing, Vol. 28, No. 3, 1990.

Pirandello, Luigi. *On Humor*. Chapel Hill, N.C.: University of North Carolina Press, 1974.

Potter, Stephen. *The Sense of Humor*. Middlesex, England: Penguin Books, 1954.

Robinson, Vera. *Humor and Health*. In J. H. Goldstein and P. McGhee, eds. *Handbook of Humor Research*. New York: Springer-Verlag, 1983.

———. *Humor and the Health Professions*. Throfare, N.J.: Slack Co., 1977.

Samra, Cal. *The Joyful Chant: The Healing Power of Humor*. San Francisco: Harper & Row, 1986.

Schachter, S., and L. Wheeler. "Epinephrine, Chlorpromazine, and Amusement." *Journal of Abnormal and Social Psychology*, 1962.

Schaller, Christian Tal. *Rire Pour Gai-Rire*. Geneva, Éditions Vivez Soleil, 1994.

Spenser, H. "The Physiology of Laughter." *Macmillan's Magazine*, 1860.

Vergeer, Gwen and Anne MacRae. "Therapeutic Use of Humor in Occupational Therapy." American Journal of Occupational Therapy, Vol. 47, No. 8, August 1993.

Wooten, Patty, ed. *Heart Humor and Healing*. Mount Shasta, CA: Commune-A-Key Publishing, 1994.

Zillmann, Dolf, et. al. "Does Humor Facilitate Coping with Physical Discomfort?" Motivation and Emotion, Vol. 17, No. 1, 1993.

———, et. al. "Eustress of Mirthful Laughter Modifies Natural Killer Cell Activity." Clinical Research, Vol. 37, No. 1, January 1989.

———, et. al. "Modulation of Human Natural Killer Cells by Catecholamines." Clinical Research, Vol. 32, No. 1, November 1984.

——— and ———, eds. *Handbook of Humor and Psychology*. Sarsota: Professional Resources Press, 1987.

Health and Humor Resources
Individuals, Organizations and Publications

Patch Adams, M.D.
The Gesundheit Institute
6855 Washington Blvd.
Arlington, VA 22213
(703) 525-8169

Alan Agins, Ph.D.
Asst. Professor of Nursing
University of Virginia, School of Nursing
McLeod Hall
Charlottesville, VA 22903-3395
(804) 924-1647

Al's Magic Shop
1012 Vermont Avenue
Washington, D.C. 20005
(202) 789-2800

Steve Allen, Jr., M.D.
8 LeGrand Ct.
Ithica, NY 19850
(607) 277-1795

physician lecturer on humor

Dale Anderson, M.D.
2982 West Owasso Blvd.
Roseville, MN 55113
(612) 484-5162

physician doing humor programs

Lee Berk
11645 Wiley St.
Loma Linda, CA 92354
(909) 796-4112

research into biochemistry and physiology of laughter, esp. neuroimmunology

Steve Bhaerman
"Swami Beyondananda"
P.O. Box 110
Burnet, TX 78611
(512) 756-2791

lectures, workshops, books, tapes

Michael Christensen
Clown Care Unit
Big Apple Circus
35 W. 35th St.
New York, NY 10001
(212) 268-2500

clowns who visit pediatric wards

Clown Hall of Fame
Museum & Gifts
212 E. Walworth
Delavan, WI 53115
(414) 728-9075

Eric de Bont
Bont's Adventures In Clown Arts
Pardoestheater, postbus 419
6800 AK Arnheim
The Netherlands

center for learning clown arts

Mouton DeGruyter
W. DeGruyter Inc.
200 Saw Mill River Rd.
Hawthorne, NY 10532

publishes *Humor*

Glenn C. Ellenbogen
Wry-Bred Press, Inc.
10 Waterside Plaza
New York, NY 10010
(212) 689-5473

1985 published Director of Humor
magazines and organizations in
America and Canada

Fellowship of Merry Christians
Cal Samra
P.O. Box 895
Portage, MI 49081

network of Christian humorists
publishes "The Joyful Noiseletter"

Laura Fernandez
Die Clown Doktoren,
Klaren Thaler Str. 3
65197 Wiesbaden
Germany
0611-9490981

clown created hospital clown units in
Germany

William Fry
156 Grove Street
Nevada City, CA 95959
(916) 265-5125

physician researcher on humor

Cathy Gibbons
Fun Technicians
P.O. Box 160
Syracuse, NY 13215
(315) 492-4523, fax 469-1392

Laughmakers Magazine

Leslie Gibson, R.N.
The Comedy Connection
323 Jeffords St.
Clearwater, FL 34617
(813) 462-7842

lectures and creates hospital humor
carts

Lee Glickstein
Center for the Laughing Spirit
288 Juanita Way
San Francisco, CA 94127
(415) 731-6640

Art Gliner
Humor Communications
8902 Maine Avenue
Silver Spring, MD 20910
(301) 588-3561

lectures/workshops

Annette Goodheart
P.O. Box 40297
Santa Barbara, CA 93103
(805) 966-4725

laughter therapist, lectures & workshops

Joel Goodman
The Humor Project
179 Spring Street, Box L
Saratoga Springs, NY 12866

qrtrly. newsletter "Laughing Matters," lectures, workshops, annual
humor conference

Christian Hageseth, M.D.
1113 Stoneyhill Dr.
Ft. Collins, CO 80525

psychotherapist doing humor
    programs

Ruth Hamilton
Carolina Health and Humor Assn.
5223 Revere Rd.
Durham, NC 27713
(919) 544-2370

newsletter, workshops

International Humor Institute
32362 Saddle Mt. Road
Westlake Village, CA 91361
(818) 879-9085

International Laughter Society
16000 Glen Una Dr.
Los Gatos, CA 95030
(408) 354-3456

Steve Kissel
1227 Manchester Avenue
Norfolk, VA 23508-1122
(804) 423-3867

Alan Klein
The Whole Mirth Catalog
1034 Page Street
San Francisco, CA 94117

catalog of books and toys

Karen Lee
The Laughter Prescription
7720 El Camino Real B-225
Carlsbad, CA 92009
(800) RxHUMOR

Paul McGhee
The Laughter Remedy
380 Claremont Avenue
Montclair, NJ 07042
(201) 783-8383

researcher / lecturer

C. W. Metcalf
The Humor Option
2801 S. Remington, Suite 2
Ft. Collins, CO 80525
(303) 226-0610

workshops and presentations on humor

Jeff Moore
Orthopedic Coordinator
Physical Medicine / Saint Paul Medical
    Center
5909 Harry Hines Blvd.
Dallas, TX 75235
(214) 879-3848

entertains patients

Jim Pelley
Laughter Works
P.O. Box 1076
Fair Oaks, CA 95628
(916) 863-1593

workshops, newsletter

Dr. Karen Peterson
1320 S. Dixie Hwy.
Coral Gables, FL 33146
(305) 662-2654

Caroline Simonds
Le Rire Medecin
75 Avenue Parmenitier
7509 Paris, France
42-58-39-91

French version of clown care units

Dhyan Sutorius, M.D.
Secretariat of the Center In Favor of
    Laughter
Jupiter 1008
NL-1115 TX Duivendrecht, Holland
31-0-20-690028

Christian tal Schaller
15 Francois Jacquier
CH1225 Chene-Bourg, Geneva
Switzerland

Tumor Humor
Uniquest
P.O. Box 97391
Raleigh, NC 27624

Lex Van Someren
Batstangveien 81
3200 Sandefjord, Norway
034-59644
"The Mystic Clown," teacher of
   workshops

Joan White
Joygerms
P.O. Box 219, Syracuse,
NY 13206
(315) 472-2779
spreader of good cheer, resources

Patty Wooten, R.N.
"Nancy Nurse"
P.O. Box 4040
Davis, CA 95617
(916) 758-3826
author of *Humor, Heart & Healing*

Death and Pain

Personal Accounts

Alexander, Victoria. *Words I Never Thought to Speak: Stories of Life in the Wake of Suicide*. New York: Lexington Books, an Imprint of Macmillan, Inc., 1991.
Baier, Sue, and Mary Zimmeth. *Bed Number Ten*. New York: Holt, Rinehart and Winston, 1985.
Beauvoir, Simone de. *A Very Easy Death*. New York: Pantheon Books, 1965.
Broyard, Anatole. *Intoxicated By My Illness and other Writings on Life & Death*. New York: Clarkson/Potter Publisher, 1992.
Gunther, John. *Death Be Not Proud*. New York: Harper & Row Perennial Library, 1949.
Humphrey, Derek. *Jean's Way*. Los Angeles: The Hemlock Society, 1984.
———. *Let Me Die Before I Wake*. Los Angeles: The Hemlock Society, 1981.
Huxley, Laura. *The Timeless Moment*. Millbrae, Ca, Celestial Arts, 1975.
Robinson, Jess. *The Best We Could Do*. Published by author, 1982.
Rollin, Betty. *Last Wish*. New York: Simon & Schuster, Linden Press, 1985.
Ryan, Cornelius, and Kathryn Morgan Ryan. *A Private Battle*. New York: Fawcett Popular Library, 1979.
Selzer, Richard. *Raising the Dead: A Doctor's Encounter with His Own Mortality*. New York: Penguin Group, 1993.

Practical

Bausell, R. Barker, Michael A. Rooney, and Charles Inlander. How to Evaluate and Select A Nursing Home. Reading, Mass: Addison-Wesley, 1983.
Buckman, Robert, M.D. *How to Break Bad News: A Guide for HealthCare Professionals*. Baltimore: The John Hopkins University Press, 1992.

Calahan, Daniel. *The Troubled Dream of Life: Living with Mortality*. New York: Simon and Schuster, 1993

Covell, Mara. *The Home Alternative to Hospitals and Nursing Homes*. New York: Holt, Rinehart & Winston, 1983.

Doress, Paula Brown, Diana Laskin Siegal, et al. *Ourselves, Growing Older*. New York: Simon & Schuster, 1987.

Duda, Deborah. *Coming Home: A Guide to Dying at Home With Dignity*. New York: Aurora Press, 1987.

Feinstein, David and Peg Elliott Mayo. *Rituals for Living & Dying: How We Can Turn Loss & the Fear of Death into an Affirmation of Life*. San Francisco: Harper San Francisco, 1990.

Gamzales-Crussi, F. *The Day of the Dead and Other Mortal Reflections*. Orlando: Harcourt Brace and Co., 1993.

Hale, Glorya, ed. *The Source Book for the Disabled*. New York: Paddington Press, 1979.

Hill, Patrick T. and David Shirley. *A Good Death: Taking More Control at the End of Your Life*. Reading, Mass.: Addison-Wesley Publishing Co., Inc., 1992

Kramer, Herbert and Kay. *Conversations at Midnight: Coming to Terms with Dying and Death*. New York: William Morrow & Company, Inc., 1993.

Lang, Susan S. and Richard B. Patt, M.D. *You Don't Have to Suffer: A Complete Guide to Relieving Cancer Pain for Patients and Their Families*. New York: Oxford University Press, 1994.

Larue, Gerald A. *Euthanasia & Religion: A Survey of the Attitudes of World Religions to the Right-to-Die*. Los Angeles: The Hemlock Society, 1985.

Levine, Stephen. *Healing into Life and Death*. New York: Doubleday, 1987.

Lifchez, Raymond, and Barbara Winslow. *Design for Independent Living: The Environment and Physically Disabled People*. Berkeley: University of California Press, 1979.

Lorimer, David. *Whole in One: The Near Death Experience and the Ethic of Interconnectedness*. New York: Penguin Group, 1990.

Nuland, Sherwin B. *How We Die: Reflections on Life's Final Chapter*. New York: Alfred A. Knopf, 1993.

Palmer, Greg. *The Trip of a Lifetime*. New York: HarperCollins, 1993.

Philosophical

Anthony, Nancy. *Mourning Thoughts: Facing a New Day After the Death of a Spouse*. Mystic, Ct.: Twenty-Third Publications, 1991.

Aries, Philippe. *The Hour of Our Death*. New York: Alfred A. Knopf, 1981.

Beauvoir, Simone de. *The Coming of Age*. New York: G.P. Putnam, 1972.

Becker, Ernest. *The Denial of Death*. New York: The Free Press, 1973.

Butler, Robert N. *Why Survive? Being Old in America*. New York: Harper & Row, 1975.

Enright, D.J., ed. *The Oxford Book of Death*. Oxford: Oxford University Press, 1983.

Holbein, Hans. *The Dance of Death*. New York: Dover Press, 1971 (41 woodcuts originally published in 1538).

Keleman, Stanley. *Living Your Dying*. New York: Random House, 1974.

Krementz, Jill. *How It Feels When A Parent Dies*. New York: Alfred A. Knopf, 1981.

Kubler-Ross, Elizabeth. *On Death and Dying*. New York: Vintage Books, 1969.

Larue, Gerald A. *Euthanasia and Religion*. Los Angeles: The Hemlock Society, 1985.
Levine, Stephen. *Who Dies?* New York: Anchor Books, 1982.
Lewis, C.S. *The Problem of Pain*. New York: Macmillan Publishing Co., 1974.
Mitford, Jessica. *The American Way of Death*. New York: Simon & Schuster, 1963.
Moody, Raymond. *Life After Life*. Harrisburg, Pa: Stackpole Books, 1982.
Portwood, Doris. *Common Sense Suicide: The Final Right*. Los Angeles: The Hemlock Society, 1978.
Quill, Timothy E., M.D. *Death and Diginity: Making Choices and Taking Charge*. New York, London: W.W. Norton and Company, 1993.
Ross, Maggie. *Seasons of Death and Life: A Wilderness Memoir*. San Francisco: Harper San Francisco, 1990.
Sivananda, Sri Swami. *What Becomes of the Soul After Death?* India: The Divine Life Society, 1972.
Stoddard, Sandol. *The Hospice Movement*. New York: Vintage Books, 1978.
The Tibetan Book of the Dead.

Literary

Agee, James. *A Death in the Family*. New York: McDowell, Obolensky, 1957.
Albee, Edward. *All Over* (drama). New York: Atheneum, 1971.
Anderson, Robert. *I Never Sang for My Father* (drama). New York: Random House, 1966.
Bacon, Francis. "Of Death" (essay). In *The Works*. New York: Garrett Press, 1968.
Buck, Pearl S. *A Bridge for Passing*. New York: John Day, 1962.
Camus, Albert. *The Plague*. Translated by Suart Gilbert. New York: Modern Library, 1948.
Celine, Lewis-Ferdinand. *Death on the Installment Plan.*Translated by Ralph Manheim. New York: New Directions, 1966.
Clark, Brian. *Whose Life Is It Anyway* (drama). In *The Best Plays of 1978–1979*. Edited by Otis L. Guerney, Jr. New York: Dodd, Mead, 1979.
Coleridge, Samual Taylor. "Rhyme of the Ancient Mariner." In *The Poetical Works of Samuel Taylor Coleridge*. London: Macmillan, 1925.
Cristofer, Michael. *The Shadow Box* (drama). New York: Avon Books, 1977.
Dickinson, Emily. "Death Is Like the Insect." In *The Complete Poems of Emily Dickenson*. Boston: Little, Brown, 1924.
Dostoevsky, Fyodor. *Notes from the Underground*. New York: Dutton, 1960.
Everyman. In *Three Medieval Plays*. Edited by John Piers Allen. London: Heinemann Educational, 1971.
Faulkner, William. *As I Lay Dying*. New York: Random House, 1964.
Frankl, Viktor E. *Man's Search for Meaning*. New York: Washington Square Press, 1963.
Frost, Robert. "The Death of the Hired Man." In *Collected Poems of Robert Frost*. New York: Halcyon House, 1939.
Gustafsson, Lars. *The Death of A Beekeeper*. Translated by Janet K. Swaffer and Guntram H. Weber. New York: New Directions, 1981.
Kafka, Franz. *The Metamorphosis*. Translated by A.L. Lloyd. New York: Vanguard, 1946.
Millay, Edna St. Vincent. "Renascence." In *Collected Poems*. New York: Harper, 1956.
Monette, Paul. *Love Alone*. New York: St. Martin's Press, 1988.

Moore, Marianne. "What Are Years?" In *The Complete Poems of Marianne Moore*. New York: Viking, 1981.

Olds, Sharon. *The Dead and the Living*. New York: Alfred A. Knopf, 1984.

Olsen, Tillie. *Tell Me A Riddle*. New York: Dell, 1961.

Pomerance, Bernard. *The Elephant Man*. In *The Best Plays of 1978–1979*. Edited by Otis L. Guernsey, Jr. New York: Dodd, Mead, 1979.

Porter, Katherine Anne. *Pale Horse, Pale Rider*. New York: Harcourt, Brace, 1939.

Sartre, Jean-Paul. *Nausea*. Norfolk, Conn.: New Directions, 1964.

Sexton, Anne. *Live or Die*. Boston: Houghton Mifflin, 1966.

Solzhenitsyn, Alexander. *Cancer Ward*. Translated by Rebecca Frank. New York: Dial Press, 1968.

Stevens, Wallace. "Sunday Morning:" In *Collected Poems*. New York: Alfred A. Knopf, 1954.

Tolstoy, Leo. *The Death of Ivan Ilyich*. Translated by Lynn Solotaroff. New York: Bantam, 1981.

Welty, Eudora. *The Optimist's Daughter*. New York: Random House, 1972.

Wharton, William. *Dad*. New York: Alfred A. Knopf, 1981.

Whitman, Walt. "Out of the Cradle Endlessly Rocking" and "When Lilacs Last in the Dooryard Bloomed." In *Complete Poetry and Collected Prose*. The Library of America. New York: Viking Press, 1982.

Community Living

Theory

Bellamy Edward. *Looking Backward*. Boston: Houghton Mifflin, 1898.

Berneri, Marie Louise. *Journey Through Utopia*. Boston: Beacon Press, 1950.

Bookchin, Murray. *The Ecology of Freedom*. Palo Alto, Calif: Cheshire Books, 1978.

Butler, Samuel. *Erewhon*. Edited by William Alfred Eddy. New York: T. Nelson & Sons, 1930.

Callenbach, Ernest. *Ecotopia*. Berkely: Banyan Tree Books, 1975.

———. *Ecotopia Emerging*. Berkeley: Banyan Tree Books, 1981.

Campanella, Tommaso. *City of the Sun*. Berkely: University of California Press, 1981.

Cohen, Lottie, et al., ed. *Cooperative Housing Compendium*. Davis, Ga.: Center for Cooperatives, 1993.

Driver, Tom F. *The Magic of Ritual*. San Francisco: Harpers, 1991.

Ehrenhalt, Alan. *The Lost City*. New York: Bask Books, 1995.

Fourier, Charles. *Design for Utopia*. New York: Schocken Press.

Goodman, Paul, and Percival Goodman. *Communitas*. New York: Vintage Books, 1960.

Hanson, Claus. *The Cohousing Handbook*. Port Robert's, Wa.: Hartley and Marks Publishers, 1996.

Hinds, William A. *American Communities and Cooperative Colonies*. Chicago: Porcupine Press, 1975.

Kanter, Rosebeth Moss. *Commitment and Community*. Cambridge: Harvard University Press, 1972.

Kilpatrick, Joseph. *Better Than Money Can Buy.* Winston-Salem: Inner Search Publishing, 1995.

Kriyananda, Swami. *Cooperative Communities.* Ananda Publications.

Kropotkin, Peter. *Mutual Aid.* Boston: Extending Horizon Books, 1955.

Lasky, Melvin. *Utopia and Revolution.* Chicago: University of Chicago Press, 1976.

LeGuin, Ursula. *The Dispossessed.* New York: Harper & Row, 1974.

Mannheim, Karl. *Ideology and Utopia.* New York: Harcourt, Brace & World, 1953.

Manuel, Frank, and Fritze Manuel. *Utopian Thought in the Western World.* Cambridge, Mass.: Harvard University Press, 1979.

McNeill, William H. *Keeping Together in Time.* Cambridge: Harvard University. Press, 1995.

More, Sir Thomas. *Utopia.* Edited by J. Rawson Lumby. Cambridge, Cambridge University Press, 1956.

Morehouse, Ward, ed. *Building Sustainable Communities.* New York: The Bootstrap Press, 1989.

Morris, William. *Escape from Nowhere.* International Publishers.

Norwood, Ken, and Kathleen Smith. *Building Community in America.* Berkeley: Shared Living Resource Center, 1995.

Nozick, Robert. *Anarchy, State and Utopia.* New York: Basic Books, 1974.

Peck, Scott M. *The Different Drum: Community-Making and Peace.* New York: Simon and Schuster, 1987.

Plato. *Republic.* Edited and translated by I. A. Richards. Cambridge: Cambridge University Press, 1966.

Shaffer, Carolyn R., and Kristen Anundsen. *Creating Community Anywhere.* New York: G. P. Putnam's Sons, 1993.

Skinner, B. F. *Walden Two.* London: Macmillan, 1948.

Tod, Ian, and Michael Wheeler. *Utopia.* Glendale, Calif: Crown Publishers, 1978.

Vanier, Jean. *Community and Growth.* Mahwah, N.J.: Paulist Press, 1979.

Veysey, Laurence. *The Communal Experience.* New York: Harper & Row, 1973.

Walter, Bob, et. al., ed. *Sustainable Cities.* Los Angeles: Eco-Home Media, 1992.

Wells, H. G. *A Modern Utopia.* Lincoln, Nebr.: University of Nebraska Press, 1967.

White, Frederic Randolph. *Famous Utopias of the Renaissance.* New York: Hendricks House, 1955.

Williamson, Scott, G., and Innes Pearse. *Science, Synthesis and Sanity.* Edinburgh: Scottish Academic Press, 1980.

———. *Ecotopia Revisited.* Kanter, Rosebeth Moss. *Commitment and Community.* Cambridge, Mass.: Harvard University Pres, 1972.

Practice

Andrews, Edward. *The People Called Shakers.* New York: Dover Books, 1970.

Arnold, Emmy. *Torches Together: The Story of the Bruderhof Communities.* Rifton, N.Y.: Plough Publishing House, 1964.

Autobiography of Brook Farm. New York: Prentice Hall, Inc.

Beame, Hugh, et al. *Home Comfort: Stories and Scenes of Life on Total Loss Farm.* New York: Saturday Review Books, 1973.

Bens mann, Dieter, et al. *Das Kommune Pouch.* Göttinger: Verlag Die Werkstatt, 1996.

Burkowitz, Bob. *Local Heroes*. Lexington, Mass.: Lexington Books, 1987.

Das Europäische Projekte—Verzeichnis 97/98. *Eurotopia: Leben in Gemeinschaft*. Beinin: Bezug: Eurotopia, 1997.

Duberman, Martin. *Black Mountain*. New York: E. P. Dutton, 1972.

Fairfield, Richard. *Communes USA: A Personal Tour*. Baltimore: Penguin Books, 1972.

Fitzgerald, Frances. *Cities on a Hill*. New York: Simon and Schuster, 1986.

Fogarty, Robert. *The Righteous Remnant*. Kent, Ohio: Kent State University Press, 1981.

Gaskin, Stephen. *Volume One*. The Book Publishing Company, Summertown, TN 38483.

Gravy, Wavy. *The Hog Farm*. Links Books.

Haggard, Ben. *Living Community: A Permaculture Case Study*. Santa Fe: Sol y Sombra Foundation, 1993.

Hermann, Janet Sharp. *The Pursuit of a Dream*. New York: Oxford University Press, 1981.

Hine, Robert. *California's Utopian Colonies*. Berkeley: University of California Press, 1953.

Holloway, Mark. *Heavens on Earth: Utopian Communities in America 1680–1880*. New York: Dover Books, 1951.

Hostetler, John. *Amish Society*. Baltimore: Johns Hopkins Press, 1968.

Houriet, Robert. *Getting Back Together*. New York: Coward, McCann & Geoghegan, 1971.

Institute for Community Economics. *The Community Land Trust Handbook*. Emmaus, Pa.: Rodale Press, 1982.

Interaction Member Profiles 1993. Washington D.C.: Interaction, 1993.

Janzen, David. *Fire, Salt, and Peace: Intentional Christian Communities Alive in North America*. Evanston Il.: Shalom Mission Communities Press, 1996.

Kagan, Paul. *New World Utopias*. New York: Penguin Books, 1975.

Kerista Commune. *Kerista*. Performing Arts Social Society, 1984.

Kinkade, Kathleen. *A Walden Two Experiment*. New York: William Morrow & Co., 1973.

Kinkade, Kat. *Is It Utopia Yet?* Louisa, Va.: Twin Oaks Press, 1994.

Kipps, Harriet Clyde, ed. *Volunteerism: The Directory of Organizations, Training, Programs and Publications*. New Providence, New Jersey: R.R. Bowker, 1991.

Komar, Ingrid. *Living the Dream* (Twin Oaks Community), Norwood Editions.

Krishna, Anirudh, ed. *Reasons for Hope: Instructional Experiences in Rural Development*. West Hartford: Kumarian Press, 1997.

Lee, Dallas. *The Cotton Patch Evidence*. New York: Harper & Row, 1971.

Lockwood, George. *The New Harmony Movement*. New York: D. Appleton and Co., 1905.

MacCarthy, Fiona. *The Simple Life, C.R. Ashbee in the Cotswolds*. Berkeley: University of California Press, 1981.

McCamant, Kathryn, and Charles Durett. *Cohousing—A Contemporary Way of Housing Ourselves*. Berkeley: Ten Speed Press, 1988.

McKee, Rose. *Brother Will and the Founding of Gould Farm*. William J. Gould Assoc., 1963.

McLaughlin, Corinne and Gordon Davidson. *Builders of the Dawn*. Walpole, N.H.: Stillpoint Press, 1985.

Metcalf, Bill. *From Utipian Dreaming to Communal Reality: Cooperative Lifestyles in Australia*. Sydney: UNSW Press, 1995.

Melville, Keith. *Communes in the Counter Culture*. New York: William Morrow & Co., 1972.

Mintz, Jerry, Raymond and Sidney Solomon. *The Handbook of Alternative Education*. New York: MacMillan Publishing Co., 1994.

Nordhoff, Charles. *The Communistic Societies of the United States.* New York: Schocken Books, 1965.

Noyes, John Humphrey. *Strange Cults and Utopias of 19th Century America.* New York: Dover Books, 1969.

Pearse, Innes H. *The Peckham Experiment.* London: Allen & Unwin, 1943.

Peters, Victor. *All Things Common, The Hutterite Way of Life.* Minneapolis: University of Minnesota Press, 1965.

Pitzer, Donald, ed. *America's Communal Utopias.* Chapel Hill: The University. of North Carolina Press, 1997.

Shearer, Ann. *L'Arche.* St. Paul, Minn.: Daybreak Press, 1975.

Spiro, Melford. *Kibbutz: Venture in Utopia.* New York: Schocken Books, 1970.

Sundancer, Elaine. *Celery Wine: Story of a Country Commune.* Community Publications Cooperative, 1973.

Taylor, James B. *Mary's City of David.* Benton Harbor, Mi.: Mary's City of David Publishing, 1996.

Weisbrod, Carol. *The Boundaries of Utopia.* New York: Pantheon Books, 1980.

Whyte, William, and Kathleen Whyte. *Making Mondragon.* New York: Cornell University Press, 1988.

Williams, Paul. *Apple Bay.* New York: Warner Books.

Yablonsky, Lewis. *Synanon.* Baltimore: Pelican Books, 1965.

Zablocki, Benjamin. *The Joyful Community.* Baltimore: Penguin Books, 1971.

Leadership and Power

Burns, James MacGregor. *Leadership.* New York: Harper and Row, 1978.

Canetti, Elias. *Crowds and Power.* New York: Continuum Press.

Center for Applied Studies. *The Servant as Leader.* 17 Dunster St., Cambridge, MA 02138.

Kriyananda, S. *The Art of Creative Leadership.*

Schmookler, Andrew Bard. *The Parable of the Tribes.* Berkeley: University of California Press, 1984.

Sennett, Richard. *Authority.* New York: W.W. Norton, 1986.

Cultural Transformation

Capra, Fritjof. *The Turning Point.* New York: Simon & Schuster, 1982.

———, and Charlene Spretnak. *Green Politics.*

Drengson, Alan. *Shifting Paradigms.* Lightstar Press.

Ferguson, Marilyn. *The Aquarian Conspiracy.* Los Angeles: J. P. Tarcher Publishing, 1980.

Fuller, R. Buckminster. *Utopia or Oblivion.* New York: Bantam Books, 1969.

Katz, Michael, ed. *Earth's Answer.* New York: Harper & Row, 1977.

Smuts, General Jan. *Holism and Evolution.* Greenwood Press.

Thompson, William Irwin. *Passages About Earth.* New York: Harper & Row, 1973.

———. *At the Edge of History: Speculations on the Transformation of Culture.* New York: Harper and Row.

Periodicals

Building Economic Alternatives, Coop America. 2100 M Street, N.W. Washington, DC 20063
Communal Societies, Center for Communal Studies, Univ. of S. Indiana, Evansville, IN 47712
Communities—A Journal of Cooperative Learning. 105 Sunset Street, Stelle, IL 60919.
In Context—A Quarterly of Humane Sustainable Culture. P.O. Box 2107, Sequim, WA 98382.
Kerista: Journal of Utopian Group Living. Kerista Publications / Performing Arts Society.
New Opinions, Mark Satin, Editor. 2005 Massachussetts Avenue, N.W., Washington, DC 20063
Whole Earth Review P.O. Box 38, Sausalito, CA 94966

Directories

A Guide to Cooperative Alternatives. Community Publications Cooperative. 105 Sun Street, Steele, Il 60919.
Alternative Communities. The Teachers. 18 Garth Road, Bangor Gwynedd, North Wales.
New Age Directory. Victor Kulvinskas. Omangod Press.

Building and Land Planning

Alexander, Christopher. *A Pattern Language.* New York: Oxford University Press, 1977.
———. *The Production of Houses.* New York: Oxford University Press.
———. *The Timeless Way of Building.* New York: Oxford University Press, 1979.
Alternatives in Energy Conservation: The Use of Earth Covered Buildings. Proceedings of a Conference funded by the National Science Foundation. Washington: National Science Foundation, 1975.
Ardalan, Nader, and Lateh Bakhtiar. *The Sense of Unity, The Sufi Tradition in Persian Architecture.* Chicago: University of Chicago Press, 1973.
Besset, Maurice. *Le Corbusier: To Live in the Light.* New York: Rizzoli International Pub., 1987.
Bloom, Alan. *Perennials for Your Garden.* New York: Scribner, 1975.
Bourden, David. *Designing the Earth.* New York: Harry Abrams, 1997
Bring, Mitchell, and Josse Wayenberg. *Japanese Gardens.* New York: McGraw-Hill Book Co., 1981.
Coates, Gary. *Eric Asmussen, Architect.* Stockholm: Byggfôrlaget, 1997.
de Moll, Lane, ed. *Rainbook: Resources for Appropriate Technology.* New York: Schocken Books, 1977.
Douglas, William Lake. *Hillside Gardening.* New York: Simon & Schuster, 1987.
Doxiadis, C. A. *Building Entopia.* New York: W. W. Norton & Co., 1975.
Dunne, Thomas, and Luna B. Leopold. *Water in Environmental Planning.* San Francisco: W. H. Freeman and Co., 1978.

Grabow, Stephen. *Christopher Alexander: The Search for a New Paradigm in Architecture.* Oriel Press.

Hait, John. *Passive Annual Heat Storage.* Missoula, Mont.: Rocky Mountain Research Center, 1983.

Hashimoto, Fumio. *Architecture in the Shoin Style.* Kodansha International, Ltd. 1981.

Higuchi, Tadahiko. *The Visual and Spatial Structure of Landscapes.* Cambridge: MIT Press, 1983.

Horn, Walter, and Ernest Born. *The Plan of St. Gall.* Berkleley: University of California Press, 1979.

Howard, Ebenezer. *Garden Cities of Tomorrow.* Cambridge: MIT Press, 1965.

Jeavons, John. *How to Grow More Vegetables.* Berkeley: Ten Speed Press, 1979.

Khalili, Nader. *Ceramic Houses.* New York: Harper & Row, 1986.

Labs, Kenneth, and Donald Watson. *Climatic Design.* 1983.

Le Corbusier. *Towards a New Architecture.* New York: Praeger Publishers, 1946.

Lobell, John. *Between Silence and Light.* Boston: Shambhala Publishers, 1979.

Logsdon, Gene. *Organic Orcharding.* Emmaus, Pa.: Rodale Press, 1981.

Malkin, Jain. *Hospital Interior Architecture.* New York: VanNostrand Reinhold, 1990.

———.*Medical and Dental Space Planning.* New York: VanNostrand Reinhold, 1990.

Maritinell, Cesar. *Gaudi.* Cambridge, Mass.: MIT Press, 1967.

McHarg, Ian. *Design with Nature.* Garden City, N.Y.: Doubleday, 1971.

Merrill, Richard, ed. *Energy Primer.* New York: Dell Publishing Co., 1974.

Minckler, Leon. *Woodland Ecology.* Syracuse, N.Y.: Syracuse University Press, 1975.

Mollison, Bill. *Permaculture, Vol. 1 and Vol. 2.*

Morse, Edward. *Japanese Homes and Their Surroundings.* New York: Harper, 1885; New York: Dover Books, 1961.

Phelps, Herman. *The Craft of Log Building.* Buffalo, N.Y.: Firefly Books, Ltd., 1982.

Point Foundation. *The Essential Whole Earth Catalog.* Garden City, N.Y.: Doubleday, 1986.

Price, Lorna. *The Plan of St. Gall in Brief.* Berkeley: University of California Press, 1982.

Rudofsky, Bernard. *Architecture Without Architects.* Garden City, N.Y.: Doubleday, 1964.

Safdie, Moshe. *Form and Purpose.* Boston: Houghton Mifflin Co., 1982.

———. *For Everyone a Garden.* Cambridge: MIT Press. 1974..

Schuyt, Michael, et al. *Fantastic Architecture.* New York: Harry N. Abrams, 1980.

Shelter. Bolinas, Calif.: Shelter Publications, 1973.

Simonds, John Ormsbee. *Landscape Architecture.* New York: McGraw-Hill Book Co., 1983.

Smith, Russell J. *Tree Crops.* New York: Harper Colophon Books, 1950.

Sullivan, Louis. *Kindergarten Chats.* New York: Dover Books, 1980.

———. *The Autobiography of an Idea.* New York: American Institute of Architects, 1926

The Underground Space Center. *Earth Sheltered Design.* New York: Van Nostrand Reinhold Co., 1979.

Van der Ryn, Sim. *Ecological Design.* Washington D.C.: Island Press, 1996.

Van der Ryn, Sim, and Peter Calthorpe. *Sustainable Communities.* San Francisco: Sierra Club Books, 1986.

Venolia, Carol. *Healing Environments.* Berkeley: Celestial Arts, 1988.

Wright, Frank Lloyd. *The Future of Architecture.* New York: Horizon Press, 1953.

———. *The Living City.* New York: Horizon Press, 1958.

———. *The Natural House.* New York: Horizon Press, 1954.

Periodicals

ASE (Alternative Sources of Energy), 107 South Central Avenue, Milaca, MN 56353.
Fine Homebuilding. Taunton Press, Newtown, CT 06470.
Hortideas. Route 1 Box 302, Gravel Switch, KY 40328.
Real Gods, 966 Mazzoni Street, Ukiah, CA 95482.
Tranet: Transnational Network for Appropriate Technologies. Box 567, Rangeley, ME 04970.

Art as Therapy

Csikszentmihalyi, Mihaly. *Flow: the Psychology of Optimal Experience.* New York: Harper and Row, 1990.
Dewey, John. *Art As Experience.* New York: Capricorn Books, 1934.
Koestler, Arthur. *The Art of Creation.* New York: Macmillan, 1964.
May, Rollo. *The Courage To Create.* New York: Bantam Books, 1975.
Nachmanovitch, Stephen. *Free Play.* Los Angeles: Jeremy Tarcher, 1990.
Oech, Roger von. A Kick in the Seat of the Pants. New York: Perennial Library, 1986.
———. A Whack on the Side of the Head. New York: Warner Books, 1983.

Organizations

International Arts in Medicine
Association
19 South 22nd Street
Philadelphia, PA 19103

National Coalition of Arts Therapy Associations
505 11th Street, S.E.
Washington, D.C. 20003
(202) 543-6864

International Society for Music for Medicine
Paulmannshoher Strasse 17
D-5880 Ludenscheid, Germany

Index